What Happens When you Touch the Body?

The Psychology of Body-Work.

Clive Hazell PhD and Rosalinda Perez D.N.

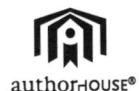

authorHOUSE®

AuthorHouse™
1663 Liberty Drive
Bloomington, IN 47403
www.authorhouse.com
Phone: 1-800-839-8640

First published by AuthorHouse   8/26/2011

ISBN: 978-1-4634-1131-2 (e)
ISBN: 978-1-4634-1130-5 (sc)

Library of Congress Control Number: 2011909232

Printed in the United States of America

C O N T E N T S

SECTION I: TRAUMA AND THE BODY

SECTION II BIOPSYCHOSOCIAL DEVELOPMENT CHALLENGES AND THE BODY

SECTION III SOCIAL SYSTEMS AND THE BODY

SECTION IV: INTERPERSONAL RELATIONS AND THE PRACTICE OF BODY WORK

SECTION V CREATING A GROWTH-FACILITATING ENVIRONMENT

DEDICATION AND ACKNOWLEDGEMENTS

We would like to dedicate this book to all the teachers and authors that have provided us with insight and information over the decades we have been interested in this field. The ideas of Leonard Hochman, Alexander Lowen, Wilhelm Reich, Robert Lewis and many others are found throughout this work. We would also like to express gratitude to the body-workers who shared their ideas and experiences with us to help bring this book to life. We hope that the inevitable errors we make in our presentation do not obscure their important messages, but stimulate curiosity in the reader to explore this important field further.

We would also like to thank the practitioners, students and clients who shared their ideas and stories with us. Also much gratitude goes to Shawna Foose who offered so much help and clarity in editing.

SECTION I:
Trauma and the Body

INTRODUCTION

It is the purpose of this book to examine the psychological side of working with the body. When body workers, massage therapists, naprapaths, chiropractors, exercise physiologists, sports trainers, work with people's bodies, they will inevitably run into many psychological factors. Many of these will be fairly clear-cut, such as a person's obvious level of motivation to change, or his/her level of comfort with his/her body. Many psychological responses involved in body work, responses that involve both the recipient and the giver of care or treatment will be quite puzzling and surprising, and may present the professional with difficulties that he/she might not have anticipated. This short text is aimed at providing some ideas that might help the body work professional to anticipate, explain and productively work with many of these less than obvious responses people have to interventions aimed at their bodies. This is a new field. Fortunately it is a growing field, for knowledge of these phenomena has great bearing on the effectiveness of treatment and on people's well being.

CHAPTER 1

Remembering With the Body

Assumptions

Before we proceed, let us forward a few assumptions that the ideas in this book are based on. We use the term "assumptions" rather than "facts" for a number of reasons. One important reason is that this is a relatively new field. New things are being discovered as this approach to the mind and the body gains ground. The field is dynamic and in a state of flux. It is our hope that this approach, an approach that truly honors the deep unity of mind and body will continue to gain ground in the decades to come. We truly believe it offers great hope and possibilities for the alleviation of human suffering. So great are these possibilities, that one has to be creative indeed in order to generate explanations as to why these ideas are not and have not been explored more vigorously. (But that is the subject of another book!)

1. We "speak" with our bodies.
The human body has many languages. In this course of study we will touch lightly on some and explore others in more depth.

When most people think of the language of the body they think of gestures and bodily positions. Birdwhistle (1975) writes of this in "Kinesics and Context". We will examine some of his ideas.

Another language of the body is less "fluid" and more structural in nature. This line of thought argues that the characteristic forms of the

1

body, its shape, posture, energy distribution, express the character of the individual. When we decode the language of the body in this way we may see the person's personality, his/her history and issues, often unconscious issues. The major exponents of this approach are Lowen (1972, 2003a, 2003b, 2005) and Reich (1933).

Our body structure is affected by many different factors: genetics, accidents, illnesses, diet, culture, personal choice and psychosocial trauma are items that would certainly be on the beginning list of forces that shape us, shape us not only emotionally, but physically. All of these interact and mix together to give us the body we have today and to give the next client we see the body they present us with.

In this study, our special focus will be on the impact of psychosocial trauma on the body and how this affects those who would work with the body.

To be an effective body-worker, it is necessary to not only listen to the patient's spoken communications. It is also essential that the practitioner listen to the languages of the body, and be aware that most of the communication that goes on between people is encoded in these forms.

This study can be regarded as a primer for the multiple forms of body languages. It is a primer because I assume that this field of study is something that we will be learning for the rest of our lives.

Link to Experience

Many people who work with the body report experiences like the following. They are palpating a muscle, or asking a patient to perform a certain action when, out of the blue, the patient has a powerful emotional reaction. They might start to cry, or become angry, for example. The patient themselves might be puzzled and frightened by their response. Often the body worker is also taken aback. The following case vignette gives an example of this:

Case Vignette: Andrew *is a healthcare worker in his mid-forties. He is married and has two children. He comes to Max, a massage therapist, complaining of plantar fasciitis. It is so bad that he cannot walk barefoot and has had to stop his exercise regimen. He is contemplating surgery. After two sessions with Max the pain has abated and he has postponed the surgery. He continues the weekly treatment for four months and shows*

*small gains. He complains that he thinks he has "restless leg syndrome".
Max is unsure of this and notes an inward rotation of the left leg, the
same side as the plantar fasciitis, and starts to work with the tibialis.
Andrew starts getting irritated. Max senses an opportunity and says, "If
you are willing we can just see where this takes us. Stay in touch with those
feelings. There isn't much I haven't seen." Andrew trusts Max enough to
give it a try and stays with the bodywork and the feelings. Andrew's leg
starts to shake a lot and Andrew, who was usually quite quiet growls in
rage and then lets out a roar. His left leg flops around and then he slams
it onto the table, after which his whole body goes limp. Max ends the
treatment with a relaxation massage. The next day Andrew calls to report
that the pain has gone completely and that he was able to start exercising
again. Max notes to himself that it is as if the plantar fasciitis contained a
lot of pent up rage. Interestingly, the source of this rage and the meaning
of the outburst on the treatment table was never addressed. Max's relief
continued unabated.*

What is happening here?

This common experience can be explained as follows. The patient
was traumatized emotionally by something in his past. He has, for the
most part, placed that trauma and the memory of it, in the repressed
part of his unconscious mind. However, there are strong isomorphisms
(parallels) between the body and emotional experience. Thus the
musculature that was involved in the trauma has become involved
in the unconscious memory of the bad experience. When the body
worker activates that muscle in a certain way, it also activates the
unconscious memory and all the connected thoughts and feelings. The
repression weakens and the feelings flood to the surface, sometimes
along with the memories of the trauma, sometimes not. It is as if, when
we work with the body we are working directly with the mind and its
mechanisms of defense. For this reason, the body worker needs to be
equipped with some basic psychological ideas. We are not arguing that
the body worker should be or become a psychotherapist (although
that could be done and in our opinion would be a wonderfully
powerful combination). What is helpful, however, is if the body worker
can understand these phenomena as they occur, provide some basic
empathy and understanding for clients, and, if appropriate, make
referrals to the appropriate professionals.

Model of Trauma

Many of the ideas in this study are based on the theory that trauma, especially psychosocial trauma is "encoded" in the body and that body workers often encounter recrudescences of these traumatic events in the course of their work. This next section will present a simplified general model of trauma and examine its many dimensions. Below is a diagrammatic representation of a model of trauma we find useful.

General Model of Trauma

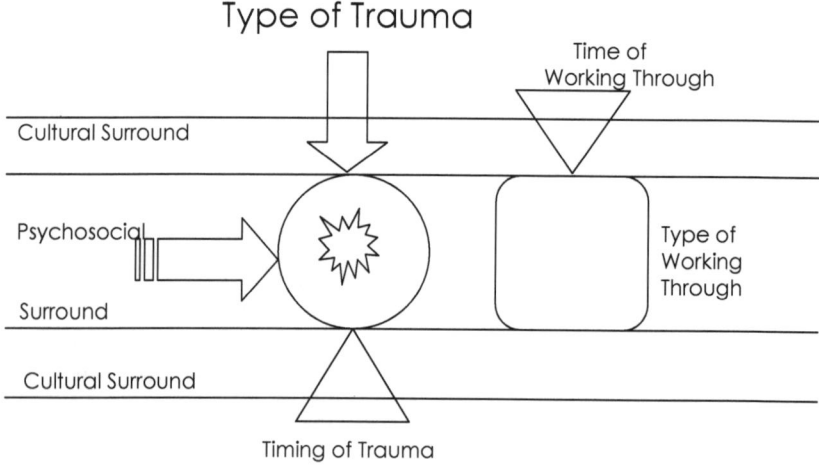

Key to Model

This model is an extremely simplified version of psychosocial trauma, but it does alert the practitioner to key elements. Following is an explanation of each of the elements in the model.

The Trauma: As we will soon see, trauma can vary along many dimensions. It can come from different sources, human or non human. It can be sudden or gradual, expected or unexpected. It can be acute or chronic. It can involve physical or psychological violence or both. It can come from those we trust or strangers. All of these variables and more will determine the intensity and seriousness of the trauma.

The Person: The individual who experiences the trauma can vary widely along many dimensions. They might be very resilient or more vulnerable. They could be outgoing and extroverted, or shy and introverted. They may have a history of serious previous traumas or not. They might be suffering from depression before the trauma occurs or be in good spirits. All of these variables and more will affect the impact of the trauma on the person.

The Timing: Traumas that occur earlier in life are usually, other things being equal more serious in their consequences than those that occur later, when people are usually better prepared to protect themselves and get help. Also we need to consider the developmental stage of the person at the time of the trauma. What psychosocial tasks were they working on that might have been derailed by the trauma, perhaps causing secondary problems?

The Immediate Psychosocial Surround: Trauma can be ameliorated or worsened by the family or circle or community one inhabits. Some of these environments can be extremely helpful in coping with and working through trauma in that they provide help, guidance and support. In other cases this support is not available and the impact of the trauma is greater.

Cultural Factors: Certain cultural factors can operate to help individuals cope with trauma. In some cultures it is customary to rely on others for assistance, while in others people are more likely to have to deal with trauma on their own. Sometimes religion plays a vital role in helping people cope with trauma.

The Working Through: Working through means the extent to which the individual "talks through" the trauma with someone else who listens and cares. This might be a professional counselor. Generally speaking the closer this is done to the trauma, the more effective it is. Early working through of a trauma will lessen its effect.

By thinking of the trauma their clients have been through in these terms, helping professionals of all kinds will be better able to assess the depth and seriousness of the trauma. For example, if a trauma was sudden, unexpected, was early in life, involved being let down by trusted others, occurred in an unsupportive social matrix and was never worked through, then the results will tend to be on the more serious end of the spectrum. Professionals should also be aware that because individuals tend frequently to deny the impact of trauma and that "symptoms" can emerge many months, sometimes years after the trauma, people frequently do not associate their symptoms to the trauma that may have happened two years ago.

Let us now look at some of the dimensions of trauma and how it might affect the body.

Types of Trauma

Trauma affects the body. When we work with the body, we sometimes reawaken memories, in different forms, sometimes disguised forms, of these traumatic events. If we, as body workers are going to be doing this, it behooves us to know something about the nature of psychosocial trauma. It is not that we are going to become psychotherapists. However, as the front-line professional, we will need some understanding of the phenomena we are encountering, how they may affect our work and when and to whom it might be necessary to make a referral.

First, trauma can be **cumulative** or **acute.** By cumulative we mean a trauma that was repetitive, or sustained over a period of time. It may have been very gradual, like the dripping of tiny drops that build an enormous stalactite in a limestone cave. This type of trauma might include the persistent negative attitude of a parent toward a child. The child may have adapted to this both emotionally and physically and may, as an adult, still be largely unaware of its origins. Sometimes cumulative trauma does not pass under the radar. It may be long-lasting and still quite noticeable in many (though often not all) ways. For example, a violent family member who was present for a long time will perhaps cause people to make adjustments in their minds and bodies, adjustments that they are all too aware of but often would like not to think about. However, when we palpate some of the involved muscles, the memories of the years of suffering may again bubble to the surface of the mind.

Acute trauma is generally short lived but can have very strong effects on the mind and body. Examples of this include sudden losses through death or illness, violent single episodes of victimization, exposure to accidents or disasters, sudden reversals in fortune, unexpected disruptions in emotional ties and attachments to people, places, and things. Acute trauma is what people usually think of when they think of trauma. We can think of this kind of trauma as a sort of single-trial learning experience. It is as though some experiences are so powerful that we do not have to be told twice. Our bodies and minds adjust permanently or semi-permanently as if the single event could easily occur again. "Once bitten, twice shy," as the saying goes. Again, this learning is encoded in the body, on a neuro-muscular, hormonal level, even down to the secretion of peptides. When we activate certain parts of the body, we activate memories. We should not be surprised if there are flashbacks, symptoms, strong emotional responses or resistances to treatment.

The following case gives an illustration of cumulative trauma (that is, one that extended over an extended period of time). It also demonstrates the important role of family dynamics in the emergence of bodily concerns. It also anticipates the discussion of "body dysmorphia" that will occur in chapter 13.

Case: "Overweight": *Alma came to Julian, a personal trainer on the advice of a physician who felt that she could benefit greatly from an exercise routine. The work proceeded well for a few weeks until one day Alma mentioned that she was thinking of stopping. Julian pressed for the reasons and discovered that it was because a couple of friends had mentioned that she was looking good, that she had bulked up somewhat and that it suited her. Alma, far from taking this as a compliment felt that what they were really saying was that she was fat. Julian assured her that this was not the case, that her body fat was quite low and that, to his eyes, she was really benefitting from the work they were doing together. Alma then went on to share that perhaps this was related to her childhood. Her father had been quite morbidly obese when she was young and her mother, anxious lest Alma should follow in her father's footsteps, put Alma on a diet at the age of three and continued throughout her childhood and adolescence to be very concerned with her weight and appearance. Alma mentioned that she had been diagnosed, during her adolescence as "borderline anorectic". Both she and Julian could see how this childhood* *experience had led to this current juncture in her life. She had a choice; to continue her "skinny" lifestyle, which was bad for her health, but kept her internal anxious mother off her back, or continue with the training and embark on a life of physical health where she no longer lived in the shadow of her mother's unrealistic concerns. Alma had good insight, realized that her mother's anxiety did not have to so completely dominate her and that her relationship with her mother could still continue on good terms even if she did put on some weight ("good weight"). She chose to continue with the personal training.*

When evaluating the intensity of trauma, we should balance several considerations. One's sense of the strength of the trauma alone is not enough. Other factors need to be considered.

Briefly, these factors are: the personality of the person traumatized, the developmental stage the person was at when traumatized, the psychosocial surround of the person when traumatized, the nature of the trauma itself, whether or not "working through" of the trauma was attempted and the extent to which it was successful, the values structure and other sustaining forces in the person's life.

Trauma theory would take a lifetime to study and master. Here we are only aiming at a quick overview so the bodywork professional can gain an initial feel for what might be going on in a clients' mind.

The personality of the victim

Some individuals are more "resilient" than others. Many factors influence resilience, and what may crush one person may not have as radical an effect on others. We must be careful to assess this factor when assessing the extent of the trauma in a person's life. For example it appears that individuals who have had strong, reliable emotional attachments to caretakers during their infancy often show greater resilience to stressors, such as trauma.

Developmental stage

Generally speaking the earlier the trauma, the more serious its effects. The ego is not as strong in the earlier years of life and this means the individual is less able to organize, integrate and make sense of the trauma. They also might not be able to remember the trauma in the more usual "adult" ways of recollection. This might mean that it will be difficult for the victim to put the trauma into words or to have it make sense to others. Often earlier traumata result in more generalized complaints. That is, they are less localized in specific regions of the body. This has to do with the fact that it takes a few years for the human child to develop a coherent body image.

Often the trauma will interfere with whatever developmental stage the person is involved in at the time of the trauma. For example if the child is very young and coping with issues of trust, then a trauma experienced at this stage will often disrupt the achievement of the developmental task.

The Psychosocial Surround

Sometimes an individual is traumatized and they are surrounded by helpful supportive people whom they confide in and who help them. Sometimes they are left alone with the trauma. Sometimes they are made to feel guilty or are even punished for being a victim. Often times they think they are bad, or crazy. Sometimes they actually do have "psychotic-like" symptoms. Sometimes they are committed and are treated as if they are ill or genetically malformed or suffering from a chemical imbalance and no one, not even trained psychology professionals addresses the underlying cause of the trauma. Many just soldier on, suffering in silence—a silence that may be metaphorically broken when a body worker unwittingly palpates a tight-knotted muscle or prescribes a certain movement regimen. In these latter cases the individual has multiple traumas to work through. First, there is the layer of the original trauma, and then there is layering of insult added to injury of often decades of misunderstanding and mistreatment.

The Nature of the Trauma Itself

Trauma varies widely in its qualities. It can be sudden, unexpected or slowly evolving and anticipated; it can involve physical or psychological violence; it can be explicit or implicit; overt or covert; acknowledged or unacknowledged; socially patterned (as with political violence) or individually-based; chaotic or organized; on and on. The clinician will gain some feel for the nature of the trauma fairly quickly and be able to empathize more effectively if they can ascertain some of its essential dimensions. This will help the person feel understood. It will help break down some of the isolation inherent in being traumatized if someone seems to understand or, at least attempt to understand, the dimensions of the experience. In addition, of course, the substantive qualities of the trauma will have an impact on the signs and symptoms of the reactions to the trauma.

Extent of Working Through

Over the past few decades, public awareness of the impact of trauma has increased so there is more likelihood of a traumatized individual receiving some treatment, either from professionals or from others. When tragedy hits, for example, a school, we frequently observe a team of counselors going in to the school in order to help the students cope with their trauma. We also acknowledge that trauma is part and parcel of armed combat. However, much trauma goes under the radar, and is unnoticed. Generally the closer to the trauma the working through is done, the easier it is. The longer you wait, the more complicated it is likely to be. When in the course of our work we encounter the re-emergence of trauma, it is important to consider the amount of working through of the trauma the individual has been able to accomplish. Is this the first time in years this person has had these memories come back? Or is this an aftershock of something they thought they had worked through, but clearly needs a little more attention? Again, awareness of this dimension is key if the healthcare professional is to offer appropriate empathy, understanding and referrals. Van der Kolk (1995, 2006) speaks of the importance of encoding the traumatic experience in language as a means of achieving some resolution of the experience. We believe that multiple language forms or symbol systems can serve this function. This would include artistic expression of all kinds, since these are symbol systems also.

Values and other Sustaining Structures

Values of various sorts have been shown to have a powerful moderating effect in the way people cope with trauma. Some people are sustained by religion, philosophy, or other values such as family, loved ones or cherished ideals and vocations. These can enable humans to do astounding things, to sustain stresses and traumata that could potentially be devastating. Again these factors must be taken into account when assessing the resilience of a person who, in the course of bodywork suffers a recrudescence of an earlier trauma. One must ask, "Does this person have a set of values and ideals that will help him/her find some meaning and support through this event?"

Perhaps, at times, there are even bodily interventions that might help activate such forces in the personality.

Transgenerational Trauma

A clinician should also be aware of the phenomenon of transgenerational trauma. Trauma can be "passed on" from one generation to another. A parent who has been traumatized may unconsciously transmit the horrible experience to their children, who, unawares, absorb it as if it was their own. This process may be especially pronounced in individuals who are more sensitive or in cultures with a higher degree of family cohesion. Thus an individual may act as if they have endured trauma, and manifest many of its symptoms while in their lives they have been relatively free of bad experiences. Upon investigation one might find that their parents or their grandparents went through traumatic experiences. Some psychologists argue (and we are inclined to agree with them) that one must sometimes go back ten generations to unearth factors causing disruptions occurring in behavior in the present. Thus, a body worker should not be surprised if a person evinces behavior as if they were traumatized when it was, in fact their forbears that endured the trauma.

Secondary Trauma/Tertiary Trauma

Often it is enough just to be a witness or a bystander to trauma to have been traumatized and to have had this experience encoded in the body. This might have happened in a family where one witnessed physical abuse or it might have occurred in one's profession where one witnessed others enduring trauma. Studies have shown that these effects can be as long-lasting as primary trauma. Often since the effects are not traced back to the traumatic experience, people are puzzled by their symptoms.

This case vignette gives an example of the re-surfacing of a traumatic experience in a patient as a naprapath worked on lower back pain. We can also see, in this story, how certain patients are able to form speedy positive alliances with the therapist and are able to "see through the pain" of some of the treatment to the relief that lies on the other side. We can also see, that when such a positive alliance or "transference," to use the psychological term, is mobilized the therapist often needs only to be warmly empathic, to be emotionally available, to listen.

Case: Hip Flexor Releases Suppressed Memories

Joline, a warm-hearted 82-year-old grandmother, came to a naprapath complaining of chronic pain in her lower back. She had lumbar vertebrae 3 and 4 fused and had this pain for at least ten years. She was taking frequent cortisone shots, and the pain kept returning.

Cindy, the naprapath, diagnosed a chronically tight hip flexor and after Joline laid down on the treatment table started to work on that area.

"That's exactly it!" exclaimed Joline. "How did you know?"

"It's a very common problem," replied Cindy.

Even after one session, the pain subsided and Joline was suffused with gratitude.

"Bless you!" she said as she hugged Cindy. As she left the office, she blew Cindy kisses through the window. It was the first time she had truly felt free of pain for ten years.

Joline returned for more treatment sessions to deepen the relief and to practice exercises to help with her posture.

As Cindy palpated Joline's hip flexors, Joline started to spontaneously talk about trauma. It was almost as if Cindy was pressing a button that released the memories and her talk. Cindy simply listened as Joline spoke about her mastectomy and traumatic childhood memories she had at the hands of her father. Cindy had the strange fleeting impression that these two events were connected in Joline's mind.

Cindy anticipated that the pain would return if not treated vigorously and so Joline returned for two or three sessions a week with work focusing mostly on the hip flexors.

As is often the case, there was a good deal of sensitivity to touch in the hip area, but Joline was adamant. "I don't care how much it hurts, honey, you keep on doing it."

Cindy pondered how some of her patients were very able, as was Joline, of tolerating the pain. With other patients, who seemed to have a low tolerance for pain, it was much harder to establish the type of working alliance she had with Joline.

This case demonstrates several important concepts. First it

illustrates the fact that many traumatic memories are "stored" as it were, in the pelvic region and that this area carries a terrific emotional burden for many people. Second, it shows the importance of language, in this case, verbalization, in the resolution of both the trauma and the physical difficulty. We also note in this case the idea of the "working alliance" between Cindy and Joline and how important this was in the working through process. The working alliance depends on emotional contact and psychological safety, among many other factors. Cindy was able to provide these and, thankfully, Joline was able to utilize them. This was enabled by the "positive transference" that Joline formed with Cindy and that enabled Cindy to maintain a therapeutic effect. Finally, we see exemplified in this case the importance of listening, pure and simple (or perhaps not so simple).

Sometimes the recollection is spontaneous and straightforward, but nevertheless, extremely useful, as the following snapshot illustrates:

Case Vignette: Castaway: *Tara, a naprapath, starts to work on Bill's tight psoas, which she believes is connected with his chronic lower back pain associated with disc protrusions at L3, 4. As she starts, he exclaims, "Do you think this might have anything to do with the fact that I spent two years in a cast as a kid?"*

CHAPTER 2

Typical Body Reactions to Psychosocial Trauma and Stress

Many writers and thinkers in this area have enumerated frequently occurring patterns of bodily reactions to psychosocial stress. Following is a brief synopsis of some of these. If the body-worker is equipped with these, perhaps they will be better prepared for some of the emotional reactions they encounter in the course of their work. The list includes:

Bracing
Encapsulation
Floppiness
Dissociation
Freezing
Contraction/Compression
Character Armoring
Energy Blockages
Reactions to touch
Splitting
Scattering
Reactions to Body Positioning
Restrictions in Breathing
Reactions to Different Bodily Zones

Bracing: Moshe Feldenkrais, in his "The Body and Mature Behavior" (2005) argues that when we are under stress or at risk we engage an

15

automatic response, a reflex, which he calls bracing, where we tense up along our spine as if to prepare for some shock to our body. He says that we can see this from the earliest days of life, as infants brace themselves when they feel insecure, perhaps when they sense they are not being securely held by their caregivers. This bracing, since it focuses so much in the spine, and since the spine is involved in a multitude of bodily and psychosocial functions, can have serious effects on the person's further adaptation to life.

Clearly, many body workers focus on the muscles around the spine. In so doing they are possibly intervening on a bodily level to "muscle memories" of trauma or stress, some of these occurring very early in a person's life.

Encapsulation: This term is derived from the work of Frances Tustin, who noticed that when individuals engaged an autistic-like defense against trauma, they would sometimes become physically like a crustacean. They would live as though they were inside a shell that protected them. Thus, in addition to Feldenkrais's bracing, we may hypothesize that some people create a hard shell with their musculature, a hard shell that, in fantasy, protects them from painful experience. Of course such a hard shell also cuts them off from many exchanges with the world—exchanges that could be enriching and sustaining.

Again, body workers may encounter such defenses in the line of their work, as they meet with strong resistances to or strong reactions to the palpation of even superficial muscles.

Floppiness: This idea is also taken from the work of Frances Tustin (1972) who noticed that some children responded to stress by just going all floppy and loose, so floppy that they would seem to merge with the person or thing they were next to. She hypothesized that this too was a way of protecting themselves. Perhaps these children felt that if they become someone or something else they would be safe. The "amoeboid" response to stress or trauma is a way of merging with another, a way of simply disappearing into the background, of perhaps, ceasing to be. Such a response, if used too much, can obviously impair the extent to which a person will be able to assert himself or herself and exercise initiative in the world.

Again, body-workers frequently will give individuals assignments that involve tensioning or activating their body or parts of their body.

If the person is engaging this type of response to some stress in their lives, then the body worker will encounter some form of resistance or anxiety in the way the patient responds to these exercises.

Frequently, the anxiety, or resistance to such an activity is not at all obvious, and may pass under the radar of the practitioner, or be categorized as something else. The client may simply not show up for the next session, sometimes giving a plausible reason. The client may develop a condition of some sort that prevents them from doing the activity. The client may become angry or display some other disturbing emotion that, at first blush, is hard to explain. However, with some of the insights in this book, the body worker may be able to provide sufficient empathy and support to assist the patient in taking the next step.

Dissociation: This is written about in fine evocative detail by Herman (1992) and is witnessed in the video, "Childhood Trauma, the Long Term Effects" (1995) Another term for this might be splitting off. It is very common for people, when they are under stress to "jump out of their skin" or be "literally beside themselves". When we are under stress, or in pain, it is a common self-protective measure to simply not be in one's body. Sometimes we activate this defense by dint of will. We make it happen, for example when we go to the dentist and have a root canal. Sometimes, however, it can be activated and be continued without our even knowing it. We become "disembodied". Alexander Lowen writes beautifully of disembodiment in "The Betrayal of the Body", as does D.W. Winnicott in many of his works(1960, 1964,1965a,1965b,1971a,1971b). R.D. Laing, in "The Divided Self" (1969) gives an excellent feeling for this psychophysical state.

We learn and relate to others, the world and ourselves through our bodies. We learn how to take care of our bodies by being in touch with them, by being in them. When we become disembodied, we again gain a reduction in pain; we survive, but at a cost to our relatedness and our vitality. Life can feel very empty if we are not at one with our bodies.

Interestingly one can often find this disembodiment in people who have taken up professions that have to do with the body—dancers, athletes, body workers.

When we work as body workers with an individual who has taken up this unrelated posture toward their body we may encounter several telling phenomena. Perhaps the person will have difficulty labeling bodily experiences or identifying where they come from. Perhaps the person will endure terrific pain and not tell you that they are experiencing it. Perhaps they will become anxious as you work with them and help them regain contact and ownership of their once disowned body. As people reclaim their body, they are likely to recall or perhaps re-experience (often in a disguised form) the very reason why they disowned their body in the first place. The body worker should anticipate and be ready for these types of responses.

Freezing: Human beings, when exposed to stress and trauma, engage what is known as the "fight, flight, freeze" response. It is an automatic bodily reaction that prepares the organism for danger. It prepares the organism to fight an enemy, flee from a threat, or simply freeze, staying perfectly still until the danger has passed. This is the response people refer to as "the deer in the headlights" reaction. We are shocked, and we become immobile. This type of response is seen quite frequently in persons who have been traumatized. Their motility or degree of bodily movement can become seriously restricted. Sometimes the whole body is involved; sometimes only sections of the body are affected—often times the sections that were involved in a meaningful way in the original trauma. For example, we have worked with clients who were seriously neglected during the first year of their lives and encountered a very hostile attitude from their mothers, especially in regard to feeding. In traditional psychoanalytic parlance, one would say that they were "orally deprived". This would show up in sessions in a characteristic pale, frozenness around their lips and surrounding mouth area. This paleness would accentuate as they encountered more stresses in their lives or in their relationships. As another example, it is also fairly common for individuals who have been sexually abused to find it difficult to have sexual feelings in their body. It is as if memories of the trauma have been frozen by their numbing the associated parts of their body. A man we once worked with was frequently hit about the head by his father. This man had frozen his shoulders in a chronically stiff self-protective position.

It is easy to imagine what might happen with these people if one were to work with their bodies and to "loosen up" or activate these affected areas. In fact as a professional or even as a friend, one often has the impulse to want to "warm up" such individuals. We perhaps should use caution. A metaphor works quite well here. If as a child you have gone into the snow to play snowballs without gloves (bare hands make the best snowballs) you know that while there may be some initial pain, eventually your fingers become numb and there is no pain. One learns from experience, however, if you warm your hands too quickly, say, by putting them under a tap of warm water, the resultant pain can be excruciating. It is far better to warm your fingers up slowly, almost unnoticeably. That way it does not hurt.

The same goes, in our experience, for frozen parts of the body, especially if they are frozen because of a psychosocial trauma. As the body "melts" so the pain comes to the surface. It is essential that there be someone there to empathize with this pain as it is essential that the pain emerge in packages that are not overwhelming to the individual's ego. Again, many factors come into play in determining how capable a person is in processing trauma.

Contraction/Compression: Sometimes when an individual is exposed to stress or trauma, they have the bodily reaction of compression or contraction. It is almost as if the entire body retracts into itself and becomes dense and tight. This organic response can be seen in life forms like the amoeba which when it encounters a noxious stimulus retracts into itself or when a slug or leech compresses itself in response to pain or danger.

Much body work is aimed at helping individuals become more expansive. Massage, for example promotes a flow of body energies (blood, awareness) to the surface, to the skin and is aimed at facilitating relaxation and expansion of tight constricted, contracted muscles. If this is done with an individual who has adopted the self-protective measure of contraction, it is likely to evoke several responses. Initially, the patient may experience anxiety as his/her characteristic life posture or stance is being undermined. The memories of the original trauma may emerge into the borders of their awareness. They may resist the treatment in some way, especially if it is too much, too soon for them. They may even seek to sabotage gains that are made in treatment by going out after the successful session and not only not following through on the body-worker's recommendations, but actively sabotaging them by engaging in activities that reverse the gains made in the treatment. Clearly, a deeper understanding of the motivations behind the patient's resistance will help the professional body worker empathize and adjust his/her treatment rather than get angry with or critical of the patient.

Character Armor: This concept was developed by Wilhelm Reich in his book "Character Analysis" (1935). Reich's idea was that when individuals suffer a trauma, they respond defensively, not only by forming psychological defenses, but also by forming what he called character armor, muscles that tightened and become hardened so as to protect one from painful emotions. Reich's theory was that this armor seriously interfered with one's sexual happiness and therefore with one's enjoyment of life in general. He felt it lead to attitudes of despair, hopelessness, misery, envy and aggression.

Reich believed that character armor didn't just occur randomly throughout the body. He believed there was a definite pattern and rationality to the way in which the tight muscles organized themselves. People with sexual traumata would show tight musculature in the pelvic area, people with issues around feeding would show tightness in the mouth area; people with issues about independence would show tightness in muscles that had to do with movement and locomotion; people who had traumata related to self expression might show tension in muscles around the voice box and so on. We examine this somewhat later on, but the notion of character armor can be very useful to the body worker, who, once they understand that tight muscles may serve the function of protecting their patient from experiencing emotional pain, may be able to better understand the meaning of some of their patients' reactions. The body worker is not only helping muscles relax; he/she may also be removing character armor. When people remove their armor, they certainly feel lighter and freer to move, but they also feel more vulnerable.

Forms of Armor: Reich noticed that character armor came in a number of definable forms. Again, we will examine this later and I refer you to the works of Reich and Lowen cited at the end of this text for further details. However a few words are useful here. Armor can occur in bands or belts around the body at key zones. Often armor forms in a belt around the mouth and base of the head, around the neck, the shoulder girdle, the diaphragm and the pelvic girdle. Each band of armor is associated with a different type of traumatic situation and a different personality type. Sometimes only one belt might be very active, sometimes several or all. In some individuals the armoring seems to switch from one belt to another with rapidity in order to accomplish its defensive function. Sometimes the armor is like chain mail and envelops the whole body. The person who uses this type of armor is usually not rigid, constrained or compressed as is the case with bands or sheets of armor. They may appear to be quite flexible and even athletic, but they are armored nonetheless, just armored with a more flexible self-protection than a band of tight muscle. Sometimes armor occurs in sheets or slabs of tissue or tight muscle that seems to protect a particular area of the body. A person's torso, for example my be clad in masses of extra tissue, or perhaps we might see a build-up of extra muscle at the upper back and at the back of the neck, as if to protect from a blow from behind. Myers (2001/2009) in "Anatomy Trains", points out that it is muscle that leads bone and the myofascia in its structure. So frequently these tightened muscles, over the long haul, will cause the bones to develop in certain directions, and the strapping of the myofascia to tighten and loosen, leading to deep structural changes in the person's body. (Of course, we have to remember the other factors, genetic and so on, that affect bodily structure; all that is being claimed here is that psychosocial forces also play a role.)

Energy Blockages: It is frequently assumed by body workers that energy flows around the body and that this energy takes on various forms. Sometimes it is conceived of in very concrete fashions, such as the transport of blood, oxygen and nutrients around the body. Sometimes it is conceived of in more abstract fashions, such as the passage of information from one area of the body to another through neuronal connections. It is also conceived of in somewhat metaphysical forms, in such concepts as "chi" or "kundalini" or as "orgone" energy (the latter being the concept used by Wilhelm Reich, although he believed that it could be measured in very physicalistic ways). Much body work concerns itself with the redistribution of energy around the body. Perhaps the skin is charged up with a massage or ignored muscles are activated in stretching exercises or prescribed activities. Perhaps awareness is directed to areas of the body that the person does not usually think about. Perhaps through palpation of tissue, blood flow is improved and suffuses areas of the body previously deprived of nutrients. All of these involve the redistribution of energy in the body. At the other end of the equation, we note that trauma brings about a redistribution of energy in the body. A person may unconsciously withdraw energy from the area or areas of the body that were involved in the trauma. A child who was not encouraged to walk, run, jump or skip; not encouraged to be independent and enjoy their motility, may have "undercharged" legs. A person who been a victim of sexual violence may have reduced the flow of energy into their pelvic area. This reduction, by the way, may be accomplished through the institution of armoring, as was discussed in the previous section. Thus when a body worker works either with the legs or feet of the first patient or the pelvic area of the second patient, and sees for themselves how much these zones of the body are "crying out" for more energy, they may run into patient resistance to treatment, because to suffuse these areas of the body with energy is to take a risk. In the first case, the risk may be that of an imagined punishment for taking pleasure in their legs and feet, the very organs that will grant them such independence. In the second case, the flow of energy into the energy-deprived area may bring forth painful memories, even to the point of a re-experiencing of the original trauma. Body workers, knowing this likelihood, are less likely to push too far, too soon and are more likely to be understanding of patients' anxieties and "resistances" to treatment. They might be able to offer some encouragement and not take it personally when a client seems not to want what the body worker has to offer. These insights offer some understanding of why people, even when they are in obvious physical pain with the way out so clear and being offered to them, still balk and stay put.

Reactions to Touch: Ashley Montagu (1986) has written a beautiful book entitled "Touch: The Human Significance of the Skin" and in it he elaborates in very convincing ways upon this theme. The skin is vital to our survival, our development and our well-being. Because of this it is imbued with terrific psychological importance and meaning. Body workers routinely touch the skin of others and therefore activate these meanings and their importance. Again, the skin itself carries "memories" and adaptations to trauma. I recall one client who, when he went for a massage was only able to tolerate touch on his back, while he was sitting. Any further contact for him stirred up considerable paranoid ideas. And yet, he was an individual who was desperately lonely and very much in need of touch, of human contact. His personal history had taught him, however, that, much as he yearned for contact, he also feared it. This ambivalence, these mixed feelings showed up in the ways he related to his body-worker. As his therapy progressed and he started to develop the capacity to relax with others, so he was able to more fully use the services of his body worker.

When we are very, very young, we have no spoken language. All we have is the language of the body as a way of communicating our deepest and most pressing needs. Touch is a very important vehicle for knowing these needs will be met, for developing a sense of basic trust in others and ourselves. People have a need to be touched, to feel in contact with others, to feel attached. In some people this need was not adequately met in their infancy and there remains in them a deep wish to be touched in a way that they have never been touched before, to be touched in a way that will make everything alright, just as the touch of a caring mother or father can make a child feel that everything is going to be alright. While many people long for this kind of touch, it is also feared, for it carries with it many deep anxieties having to do with dependency and regression into infantile states— anxieties about sliding back into the powerful emotional frames of mind encountered in childhood and infancy.

Body workers should be aware of the deep significance of touch in their work. For the body worker, it is an everyday event, often overlooked; for their patients it can have profound psychological meaning. Body workers, understanding this, will not be so surprised by some of the emotional reactions their clients have to the simple act of being touched.

Splitting: Sometimes people respond to stress by using the defense mechanism of "splitting". In this, the individual imaginarily divides themselves into two or more pieces. The idea behind this is to separate the "good" part of their life, themselves and their world from the "bad" part. Perhaps the idea behind this is to protect the good from the bad, especially since the recent trauma has, as it were, strengthened the strength of the "bad" experiences. Many body workers (Lowen, Reich) observe that these psychological splits often show up in the body. Sometimes one side of the body, or one side of the face may look very different from the other, or one side may have a different meaning for the person than the other. Sometimes these splits show up in posture and in gait; perhaps a leg flails somewhat, or the individual keels to one side.

Of course much body-work will involve activation of and attempts to ameliorate such splits and imbalances. The body worker should be aware that these splits are often not just physiological. Sometimes they are underpinned by experiences that the individual has not been able to integrate or synthesize in his/her life. As a further example, sometimes individuals who have had parents that were radically different and not "together" in significant ways will carry this marital split in their body. It is sometimes as if one side of their body has identified with one parent while the other has identified with the other, and just as with the parents, the two cannot co-operate very well.

Scattering: Sometimes when people are traumatized, they "go to pieces" and sometimes this can show up in the body. Sometimes this is quite apparent in people who are ill coordinated, not of a piece, disintegrated in their movements. Their limbs might seem to flail around as if they do not belong to the person or they may even talk about their body as if it is composed of separate pieces, sometimes with parts of the body representing subpersonalities that were formed in the wake of trauma. (Recall that this lack of co-ordination is not caused by a physical illness that can have this effect.) Sometimes, however, the fragmentation is under wraps. Some people may endure a trauma, go to pieces, but then have the wherewithal to heal themselves, but only superficially. When they are placed under a stress, perhaps psychosocial, perhaps physical, the top layer of integration dissolves or gives way under the strain and the underlying fragmentation of the self (the bodyself) emerges and is plain to see. This latter case needs the special attention of the body worker, for they can often be taken by surprise, if they are not sensitive to this possibility.

I recall once teaching a workshop on the psychology of the body in a large university. As a routine demonstration, I had one of the professors of psychology, a very accomplished, brilliant and articulate woman in her mid thirties show the rest of the class a bioenergetic exercise called "the bow" where she was to bend backwards over a cushioned stool to open the flow of energy through the chest, neck and pelvis. It is a fairly stressful exercise, but most people usually find it "opening" and often rewarding. To my surprise, this woman became acutely confused as to time and space as she did this activity. This was not just a dizziness phenomenon, having to do with something like orthostatic hypotension (the light headedness we sometimes get when we change position). This was psychogenic and she reported being flooded with some early childhood memories. It was important to spend some time with her to help her regain her grounding, to help her focus on the rhythm of her breathing, to help her re-generate an integrated body image and be with her bodyself before she was ready to continue or return to her seat. As body workers, we must be aware that just because someone looks integrated in their body and has an integrated story to tell about their life, it does not mean that there are not layers or capsules of unintegration or disintegration that might bubble up to the surface when that person is under pressure or stress, the kind of stress that might obtain with a massage, or a stretch, or a postural analysis, or a fitness test or an exercise regimen.

Reactions to Body Positioning: The literature on body work that is approached from a psychological angle, especially the work of Alexander Lowen, is replete with examples of how bodily positions affect emotional states. For example, typically if one is working with an individual and one wishes to facilitate their coming into contact with experiences having to do with early childhood, then one would have that person lie down. The theory behind this is that in the first months of life we are unable to walk. Recreating, in the treatment, the developmentally earlier position of lying down stimulates or facilitates the re-experiencing of early infantile states. Furthermore, if the body worker or therapist is still standing, being in a superior position, the patient is much more likely to view the therapist as a power figure, perhaps confusing them in some way with an earlier parental image from their own childhood. This is called the **transference.** We will examine this concept in greater depth in the next section. It is of the utmost importance to professional helpers. In fact, it is important for almost anybody who deals with other people to understand the dynamics of transference.

Now for some people, this **regression**, this sliding back to an earlier developmental phase in relation to the therapist, might be quite pleasant and smooth. For others, who had an unpleasant or traumatic childhood or infancy, this regression will be more problematic. In extreme cases, people will simply refuse to lie down. They may not be able to explain it. They will simply say they do not like it. Others may lie down, regress, and then be taken by surprise by some of the emotions that pop into their mind when they do. The helping professional should be ready to handle these emotions empathically and make suitable adjustments. Sometimes, these reactions to bodily shifts can generate very useful information on the patient's history and offer the therapist ideas for new treatment options.

Case: Regression, "The eyes are the window to the soul." *Brie, a 50-year-old woman with a diagnosis of scoliosis, had two operations and had two rods in her back. She came to treatment but when it came time to lie down on the treatment table, she seemed to play for time, as if she did not want to. Finally she laid down on her back and as she did the body-worker noticed a fleeting glimpse of terror in her eyes. Brie looked away and could not look the doctor in the eye even when it was needed as part of the treatment. The doctor felt the deep fear strike her in the solar plexus and believed that she had just caught a glimpse of a deep feeling from Brie, a feeling perhaps related to an early trauma she had experienced. The fact that it had been communicated so powerfully and non-verbally alerted the doctor to the possibility that the trauma had been experienced very early in Brie's life.*

This vignette illustrates several ideas. First is the idea of regression and bodily position. When we ask a person to lie down, we increase the likelihood of stimulating a regression, a sliding back down the developmental continuum. The patient is liable to experience emotions and thoughts typical of an earlier time in their life. While for some people this may be a pleasant, temporary suspension of adult responsibilities, for others it may represent a frightening return to unpleasant early life experiences. This latter seems to have been the case for Brie. Still other patients, perhaps aware of the regressive tug created by lying down in the presence of the doctor will refuse to do it, simply requesting that they be treated while seated or standing.

At the other end of the spectrum, one may encounter a patient who is very ready to lie down for treatment but resists treatment options or prescriptions that involve standing up. Lowen argues that this is often encountered in individuals who perhaps did not receive enough love and support during their infancy and so wish to return to this "lying down" stage and avoid the later "standing up and walking" stage. Individuals who are like this can often be frustrating to therapists. Understanding that their "resistance" is not being done out of "spite" or "laziness" but more out of a deep unmet need for support dating back to their infancy can help the therapist be more empathic and thus more effective. Lowen would also argue that one might expect such patients to form more of a dependency relationship with the therapist, perhaps seeing them as the "mother" they feel they never had. Again, understanding the depth dynamics of these therapist-patient relationships can help us offer more effective treatment.

Restrictions in Breathing: When people are traumatized their breathing is usually affected in some way. In the acute phase of the trauma, breathing is shallow and fast. In the aftermath of the trauma, especially if the trauma is not worked through, such tensions may still exist in the diaphragm that the breathing is still affected. Lowen has written extensively on the key role of breathing in bodywork and of its importance in depression and other emotional problems.

When a body-worker does work that alters the rate, pace, depth or quality of breathing, they are likely to be impacting psychosomatic memories of trauma. As the individual deepens their breathing, the memories of the trauma, the reason the breathing pattern was interrupted in the first place, will perhaps crowd back and cause the person conscious (as opposed to unconscious) distress. A body-worker who is unaware of these connections will be surprised by seemingly negative therapeutic reactions. The body worker who is aware of these dynamics can regulate the pace of his/her work with the client and show a deeper empathy for the client's concerns. Ultimately, I would argue, they are more likely to be successful.

Breathing is the stuff of life. As we breathe, so we become more alive. Who would not want to live, fully and vibrantly? Well, quite a few people who have suffered trauma have adapted to it by going into a state of "suspended animation," almost as if they can deny that there has been a trauma if they are not fully alive. Metaphorically, this reaction is similar to the possum, when, in order to survive, it "plays dead." When body-workers provide treatment for their patients that is aimed at renewing their zest, renewing their vitality, they are certainly offering a wonderful gift, but not infrequently, it is a gift that comes with a price, and the price is the remembering of traumas that may have lead to the bodily problem in the first place.

Reactions to different bodily zones: The course of psychosomatic development is cephalo-caudal, the process of development moves from head to tail. In the infant, the first areas of the body that are under volitional control are those in the head, next comes the neck and shoulders. At about six months the child will have some control over his/her arms and hands so that he/she will be able to reach and grasp something that catches his/her interest. Toward the end of the first year, the child is usually on the verge of becoming (perhaps already is) a toddler and his/her legs and feet are beginning to be controlled. This process is important for the body worker to know, especially if we believe that in working with a specific region of the body we are opening up the possibility of re-experiencing events associated with that bodily area. A general principle that emerges from these two hypotheses is that when a body worker is working with the head and neck, he or she is more likely to evoke earlier memories than if they are working with the legs and feet. The types of anxiety will correspondingly be very different for each of these areas. Other things being equal, the ego of the child is stronger when he/she is a toddler and on his/her feet and not so strong when he/she is in the dependent position of not being able to volitionally control all of his/her body. Thus when we work with the head, neck and shoulder girdle, we may expect the manifestations of trauma, if they are encountered, to be much more "primitive" in nature, more frightening, less verbal and often more distressing. When we sit people up, or stand them up, or work on their feet, we are activating an ego that is locked into a later developmental phase, a phase when the child will have the rudiments of language and its organizing power. Consequently the anxiety evoked when working on these parts of the body will usually be less intense, more available to rational thought, and thus, less distressing to one and all. Sometimes people can "lose it" (that is, temporarily lose contact with reality) when very early traumata are activated through body work (or through other means). One way to help him regain a sense of reality is to ask him to sit up, to look you in the eye (which you meet with a friendly helpful gaze and an intention to listen) and to inform him of where he is, who you are and that you think that they touched on something frightening but it was a memory, he is safe now.

Almost everybody has a "hot spot" on his or her body. Sometimes the hot spot is quite uncomplicated. For example, Ted may have broken his fibula playing rugby in his teens. Decades later it is still sensitive. Touch it the "right" way and he will jump. Other times, the hot spot is more complex in nature. Individuals who have been physically abused or sexually abused are often extremely sensitive to touch, touch in certain body areas or from certain directions. Often, individuals who have been physically abused have denied much of the impact of the abuse and are unaware of their hots pots, and are frequently unable to connect them to the trauma that they symbolize.

I recall once being in a body work workshop where a woman who had been burned on her upper chest by an enraged mother as a punishment was working with the workshop leader, attempting to remember and work through the event. He touched the upper chest area and she immediately panicked and became extremely confused. She so radically lost her sense of self-boundaries that for a while she was upset at the strange noise her body was making. It turned out to be the sound of the lawnmower outside the classroom. It took her several moments before she could regain her personal boundaries and realize that the noise was coming from outside. I have witnessed several events like this where individuals needed only a touch or a palpation of a certain muscle group to evoke a memory of a beating, being strapped down, having a tonsillectomy at an early age, receiving electro convulsive therapy, or witnessing a terrible event. These events should not, I think, prevent us from working with the body. Exactly the opposite is true, for they show us just how powerfully what are often regarded as purely "psychological" phenomena are encoded into bodily processes, sometimes for a lifetime.

This case demonstrates the association of different bodily regions with different periods in the patient's life. It also shows how body work can perhaps tap into deep areas of the person's mind, sometimes leading him/her to need extra psychiatric help.

Case: Deep Tissues and Deep Issues. Belinda *was a 30 year-old woman with a very stressful job, a job that seemed to the massage therapist to be seriously mismatched with her personality. She came to the therapist with widespread muscle pain and scheduled three sessions in three weeks. Very quickly she started to respond emotionally to the treatment. The therapist, who was used to these types of responses had warned her that this might be the case and assured her that it was ok with him. Belinda responded to the massage with growling, whimpering, crying, shaking and noises that seemed to come from deep inside her gut. These came largely in response to work the therapist did on her belly and back. The therapist encouraged*

Clive Hazell PhD and Rosalinda Perez D.N.

Belinda to stay with the feelings and demonstrated that it was ok with him by growling along with her, attuning himself as it were, to her emotional response. Belinda was mystified by these responses that seemed to come from so deep inside as they were without words and without images or ideas. Somehow, though, it felt very important for her to get in touch with them. She felt much better after the sessions; lighter and pain-free. From the perspective being forwarded in this book, Belinda was getting in touch with memories from the pre-verbal stage of her life, memories that were not encoded in verbal form but were nonetheless encoded in sensori-motor form, in her body.

Some weeks passed with no contact from Belinda. The therapist was puzzled and concerned, as phone calls were not responded to. Belinda finally showed up announcing that she had been in the hospital for six days with a "nervous breakdown." She did not go into details, but said that it was good for her and that she would like to resume treatment. The therapist noted right away that the profound responses of the earlier sessions were no more. However, when he started to work on Belinda's left leg, which had been bothering her, she had a strong emotional response that she wanted to share. She had recalled her parent's divorce when she was a little girl. She curled up like a ball outside of her parents' bedroom and slept there. She recalled that her father never seemed to notice or care about this and she was very upset at this. The therapist simply listened to this "flashback" and when ready resumed work on the leg with positive results.

What we see here again is the "storing" of memories in the body, manifesting as physical pain or symptoms. Also of interest is that the memory of the later period of life, related to the divorce, is "stored" in a part of the body that is activated later in life, namely the legs.

Belinda's life toward the end of this course of treatment showed significant changes. She changed careers, her relationship with her husband improved and they moved to another part of the country. She felt good and "more upbeat."

CHAPTER 3

Psychological Dynamisms Affecting Body Structure and Treatment Process

At the beginning of this study we examined some of the ways trauma affected the body and the different forms trauma can take. In the following section we examine some of the psychodynamics of human interaction and posit some notions on how this may show up in the course of bodywork

Introjection: When we introject something we take in the whole person (or thing or experience) into our minds. We do this unconsciously. For example, if a child is, say, physically abused by their father, one radical way of coping with this trauma is to imaginatively and unconsciously incorporate the abusive father image into one's mind. This serves as a protection because if the offending image is in one's mind then one can have more control over it; one can keep one's eye on it. Another way of thinking about introjection is that involves the complete taking in of a whole "lump" of an experience that was simply too much to handle, that could not be broken down and digested a little piece at a time. Because of its traumatic nature, it had to be swallowed whole. The eating metaphor works because we often hear people talk about how an experience gave them a lump in their throat or how they will have to spend a long time digesting a certain experience. Constrictor snakes can swallow animals whole and have their digestive juices break them down so they can become part of the living tissue of the snake. Human beings, however, do not have this function either physically or psychically. This means these undigested experiences often remain in the persons mind, active and completely or mostly unconscious for a long time. They usually have strong impacts on other areas of the person's life and behavior, often showing up in what might be called symptoms. They also will show up in people's bodies.

An introject can, in the unconscious imagination of the individual, take up residence in part of or all of a person's body. One female client we saw had a mother who hated her intensely. This client complained of chronic pain in her legs, especially her right leg. This complaint resisted the diagnostic skills of several doctors and the pain was so severe that when she first saw us she was hooked up to a small device that eased her pain by delivering mild electric pulses into her leg muscles. She could barely walk. After several weeks it became clear as we spoke of the very bad relationship with her mother some of the psychological pressure was relieved for her, so the pain in her legs reduced. This is of course, in no way proof, but is consistent with the hypothesis we are forwarding that bad relationships, especially if they occur early in life, can be introjected and take up residence in the body. As treatment continued with this client her pain continued to abate until there were significant improvements in her physical as well as her psychosocial life. She made friends, got a better job with a nicer boss, and started going on long walks as a hobby.

These thoughts, if true to any extent, could be very important for the body worker. For when a body worker is manipulating a part of a client's body or even working with his/her whole body, he/she may be, in the unconscious of the patient, interacting with an introjected person from the patient's past, and in so doing activating many memories and feelings associated with that relationship. It may even be that the bodily problem will only yield if there is some parallel counseling going on. The client I mention above was devoted to her massage therapist, who was, to her, in many ways a substitute good mother, a lifeline, a guardian angel, as well as a highly competent body worker.

Case Vignette: Sexual Abuse and Hip Flexors
Sara, 74, has hip flexors so tight that she has a stoop and cannot cross her legs. This tightness has probably contributed to arthritis. As the naprapath

starts to work on the hip flexors, Sara starts to talk about sexual abuse she suffered. The physical and emotional pain is just too deep, she claims, and asks to go very, very slowly with the treatment.

This vignette shows us the dynamism of **repression.** A split-off memory, residing in the unconscious, is surfacing as a result of the bodywork. We may also surmise that the painful relationship itself has been internalized wholesale as an introject. One might further hypothesize that as the body work continues so the memories of this painful traumatic memory will continue to resurface, placing demands on the empathic understanding of the therapist.

Repression can be thought of as forgetting something unpleasant, and then forgetting that you forgot it. On the plus side, the unpleasant memory is put out of one's conscious mind; the cost, however, is that the repressed memory continues to work in the mind (somewhat like a computer virus) and results in psychological and physical symptoms. These symptoms make no sense, seem irrational, if one is not aware of the initiating trauma, but are perfectly "rational" as one is made aware of the initiating circumstances. As some of the previous vignettes illustrate, it is often emotional trauma that is repressed, but body workers may also encounter cases like the following one, where an actual physical trauma had been repressed, only to surface in the process of body work.

Usually physical accidents are remembered, but the following demonstrates that memories of things like car accidents or falls can be repressed, too.

Case Vignette: Repressed Memory of an Accident

Peter, 45, came to the naprapath's office suffering from bilateral pain in his hips and shoulders. He even had surgery on both of his shoulders.

The naprapath formed the hypothesis that Peter had mis-alignment of posture because the pain and injury was bilateral. This led her to ask if Peter had ever had an accident, especially an accident that might have affected the sacral area. Peter replied that, no, he could not remember anything that might have caused such an injury.

Next week, Peter returned saying that he had thought a lot about what the naprapath had asked and had, to his surprise, recalled getting rear-ended in his car in his early twenties. An X-ray later confirmed that damage had been done to the sacral area, even though he recalled no pain at the time of the accident. Problems did not emerge for a few months after the crash.

We see in this story how repression can be powerful enough to block out, for a while at least, memories of even a physical trauma.

Identification: This is a natural psychological process, perhaps available to us from the earliest days of life. When we identify with someone, we take up that person's identity as if it is our own. Given that this identity is expressed in the body, this identification will show up in characteristic postures, gait, muscle tone, energy flow and so on. Often enough, when a body worker works with a patient to bring about change in a patient's body, they will be loosening the patient's identification with someone who was important to them, often a person in their childhood, often a parent. It is precisely here that the body worker can encounter problems. Many patients might feel that if they change their bodies they will be changing their identities, and also that if they change their bodies they are implicitly rejecting an identification with a parent. Many of us have been scripted with the dictum "honor thy father and thy mother" (even if we were not reared in the Christian tradition) and thus many patients will unconsciously feel that by abandoning their identification with their parent (by not having the same body as them) they are dishonoring them. Furthermore they may feel shame, fear, remorse and other forms of psychological pain at this process of dis-identification. The process of dis-identification, of becoming different in body and mind from those loved, admired (and often feared) persons from childhood is a deep lifelong process. It is a very demanding process. Body workers would be well informed to be ready for subtle, complex and intense reactions to the processes of bodily change at this deep level. This leads us to the next concept.

Resistance: It is very common knowledge that change can be difficult and challenging. New habits, new routines can threaten our equilibrium and consequently, even when the change is beneficial in some way, there is usually some part of us that will resist the change. Sometimes the resistance is quite conscious and easily observed, as when we see people go through the discomfort of breaking an addiction. Many times the resistance comes from unconscious processes. These unconscious processes can be extremely powerful and really slow down, bring to a halt or even reverse the dynamisms of change. Body workers are often in the business of facilitating change in their clients. They should therefore benefit from a basic understanding of the notion of unconscious resistance. The previous section gave us one of the multitudes of reasons why people unconsciously undermine their forward progress. They have identified with certain admired or feared people in their childhood and to change means to give up that identification. This is not an easy task. Even though its roots lie in childhood, the process of uncovering and questioning the utility of one's identifications is a lifelong task.

Envy is another powerful emotion that can undermine movement towards better health. In its obvious and conscious forms we might see an individual who resists getting better for fear of friends and family envying them their well being, and attacking them for their health. We will see examples of this in Chapter 9 of this book. Often times these attacks are not frontal attacks, but subtle and insidious in nature.

In addition, we have observed that individuals will often sabotage their own progress. If we accept the notion that each person is an ensemble of semi autonomous subpersonalities, and that these subpersonalities can interact with one another, then it would be possible for one less fortunate sub-self to be envious of a more fortunate sub-self and attack its progress or undermine its health-promoting relationship with another person. This might manifest itself in the individual picking a fight with someone to disrupt their progress, selecting friends who routinely bring them down, missing appointments, refusing to follow through on treatment plans and so on. Recall, the person is not consciously willing this self-sabotage. This is the result of the unconscious activity of an envious sub personality, a subself that probably was introjected in early childhood. (This process is much more fully explained in the section on Fairbairn's theory (1952). (See also chapter 8 of this text.) Lopez-Corvo in his excellent book, "Self Envy"(1995) also gives a fascinating account of such processes.

Fear of health and happiness is another reason people resist getting better. There can be many reasons for this to occur. One is that the state of health is a high energy, high excitation state. When we are well, we are buzzing with life, thoughts, feelings and sensations. Many people who have spent decades in depression or ill health, with lowered energy states, can at first find these high-energy states frightening, bizarre or weird. Added to this, their friends might comment on how "strange" they seem now. In reaction to this, there is a temptation, especially if there is not some helpful coaching on how to live in high energy states, to return to the duller, low energy state of sickness. In other words, there is resistance to the treatment.

Sometimes I have seen people get better, realize just what they have been doing for years and how much life has slipped by and then get filled with a painful remorse. So painful is this remorse and regret for an unlived life that they return to where they were before. This is similar to the observation made by Otto Rank (2010) that some people seem to strike a fiendish deal. It is as if they reason and say, "I am alive. If I am alive I must die. So if I do not live then I do not have to die. Therefore I will spend my life not being alive, that way I can escape the terror of death." Of course this reasoning does not make for a rich life, nor is it true, but we must remember, the unconscious is not rational in the same way that the conscious mind is.

The foregoing presents just a snapshot of some of the multitude of reasons why people resist getting well. Ouspensky (1973) wrote that the most difficult thing to get human beings to give up is their suffering. If we grasp this and the dynamics behind it, we can perhaps be more effective or at least less frustrated in our attempts to alleviate suffering.

Transference: The concept of transference has a long, complex and storied history. Here we will take its simple meaning. People will often relate to others, especially those in positions of power, as if they were their parents. It is as if we make unconscious mistakes regarding to whom we think we are relating. Consciously we think we are speaking to our spouse, teacher, friend or doctor. Unconsciously we think we are relating to mommy or daddy when we were a child. Professional helpers, by virtue of their power and importance, are especially likely to be the targets of transference. This is especially true, I believe for body workers who touch the body, the way parents might have done, who take away pain, the way parents might have done and are imbued with power, the way parents often were. The dynamic of transference can help us understand and explain many interpersonal phenomena that otherwise would be baffling. Why does a patient become so attached to you as a professional helper? Why do they get so upset when you take a week off? Why do they get so angry when you cancel an appointment? Why were they so upset when they saw you outside the office, at the beach or at a party with your family? In an ordinary egalitarian relationship these phenomena seem bizarre. But if we accept that on some level the patient has taken up the role of a child in relation to a parent, they become much more understandable and even expectable. The professional can deal with them more empathically and patiently, perhaps through the nuances of the transference learning more about the psychological life and issues of his/her patients and thus being better equipped to understand his/her struggles and even, of course, his/her bodily issues. Again, we are not suggesting that body workers become psychotherapists (although, with training, that would be a powerful mixture, we believe!). We are merely highlighting aspects of helper-patient relationships that are inevitable, so that they may be dealt with more productively. Of course, these transference phenomena will be a common experience for anyone in leadership positions—bosses, coaches, teachers, tutors and team leaders.

Countertransference: Just because one is a professional helper, trainer, healer, leader or teacher does not grant one immunity to the kinds of perceptual distortion involved in transference. There is no escaping the fact that we transfer onto all others, to a greater or lesser extent, the attitudes, feelings, fantasies, wishes, fears, hopes and thoughts that we originally aimed at our parents. This process is largely unconscious and for the most part it is benign, especially if those thoughts and feelings were positive. Sometimes, however, the healer or therapist him or herself can transfer attitudes on to his/her patients that impede progress and that undermine the task of the therapy. This is always unconscious and getting these attitudes into the conscious arena of the mind can be quite difficult and often psychologically painful. However, a true professional is willing, in our estimation, to pay this price, for the benefits are enormous in terms of increased effectiveness of his/her work with his/her patients, not to mention the peace of mind that comes with this type of training.

A simple example might help. A patient might remind the therapist of her mother, and perhaps the therapist had a hostile relationship with her mother, perhaps involving competitive feelings. The therapist offers the patient some advice and the patient asks a clarifying

Clive Hazell PhD and Rosalinda Perez D.N.

question. The therapist instead of hearing it as a question just aimed at clarifying, hears it as a challenge, as a criticism. The therapist then starts explaining herself quite forcefully, suggesting that the patient is maybe not going along with the treatment and that she should follow advice when it is sound and backed by research. Already the therapist/patient relationship is derailed and less than functional as a result of the therapist unconsciously confusing the patient with her parent.

Tomes have been written on the topic of countertransference. (See especially Racker, 1968, Searles, 1979.) It is extremely complex and subtle, but even the most rudimentary awareness of this phenomenon and one's own vulnerabilities to certain types of countertransference can help the helping professional.

The following example serves to illustrate several of the concepts touched on so far. First, it shows how dramatically and, sometimes unexpectedly, the body will "recall" earlier trauma. It also demonstrates how, at times, the body worker may be called upon to maintain emotional contact with the patient and that this is not always an easy task.

Case Vignette: An Example of Somatization:

In the video, "Trauma, the Long Term Effects" (1995), one of the victims of childhood abuse offers a very helpful example of a somatization. He reports that, as his psychotherapy progressed, he developed a troublesome and persistent cough. When he went to the doctor to have it checked out results were inconclusive. He took a course of antibiotics, but the cough persisted.

Finally, he had an insight. He recalled that as a child his mother had gotten furiously angry at him when he was swimming and that she had held his head under water for a long time. He felt that he had only been rescued by his mother's friends, who had pulled her off of him. For a long time after this incident he had a bad chest infection.

He came to the conclusion that the unexplained chest condition he was experiencing as an adult was his body's way of reminding him of this traumatic experience at the hands of his mother. He decided to talk about it and it abated.

This vignette is illustrative of several interesting and important facets of somatization. First, it is noteworthy that the somatization acts as a form of memory - an unconscious mnemonic device, serving as a means of recording certain elements of the trauma. It also appears that as the traumatized individual remembers the traumatic event consciously and utilizes other means of recording it, for example, language—speaking of the event—so the pressure to somatize decreases and the physical problem abates.

This is consistent with research (cited by Bessel van der Kolk in the aforementioned video) showing, through the use of PET scans, that when individuals were exposed to stimuli associated with their original traumas, there was a relative de-activation of the language production areas of the brain (Broca's area) and a relative activation of the right hemispheric and emotional centers of the brain. It was as if the capacity to put the emotionally charged experience of the trauma into words had been switched off. Perhaps putting the experience into words (or some symbolic form) is a key part of the process of healing. Clinical experience seems to buttress this notion. Talking through trauma seems to mitigate its negative impacts.

Often when bodyworkers are presented with this, they are placed in a quandary. Currently they usually have had little or no training on counseling or psychology. How much should they do or even attempt to do?

Perhaps, given that psychological factors are so frequently involved in physical illness and pain, more psychological training, especially basic counseling skills, such as listening, confronting, problem-solving should be included in the curriculum of body-workers. Certainly the idea of tactful referral to a psychological resource would be an important asset, and body-workers would be well advised to have close at hand a list of referrals to psychologists and counselors. They should also be sure that those counselors are not only certified and licensed, but also effective and humane. Clinical psychology is a regulated field, but the simple fact of having a degree or a license does not guarantee competence or compatibility with one's clients. Randomly skimming through the phone book is not an advisable search technique. Personal experience or word-of-mouth recommendations are more reliable sources of good referrals. It is important to know the counselor's guiding philosophy of treatment, attitudes toward pharmacological agents, experience with bodywork, clients, groups and families.

While referral may sometimes be a viable option, and may for a considerable number of patients provide an extremely effective conjunction of treatment, it may not always be possible. In these cases, the body-worker, while not veering from his/her primary task, will be able to offer some basic listening and a deep understanding based on empathy arising from a willingness to maintain emotional contact with his/her patient. Maintaining emotional contact does not necessarily imply solving the client's problems for him; it simply means that you are there with him, that he is understood, that he is not alone. In our experience, many people are so starved for empathic listening that a little goes a long way.

A vignette involving Leticia provides an example.

Case Vignette: Leticia's mother.

A body-worker noticed that every time Leticia laid down on the treatment table, she spontaneously started to talk about her relationship to her mother. Leticia, 35, was suffering from a concatenation of diffuse and mobile pains in her body, and she felt, deep down, that her mother did not love her. She experienced her mother as cold and withdrawn. The body-worker early on formed the opinion that much of the pain that Leticia was experiencing resulted from or was linked to her emotional pain she experienced in her relationship to her mother.

While the body-worker was not trained to do psychotherapy, she was able to provide empathic responses, simply showing Leticia that she heard and understood what she was saying and feeling. The body-worker was of the opinion that this, along with physical treatment, would alleviate Leticia's suffering. Indeed, within a few sessions, Leticia showed and maintained good progress.

Emotional Contact

If this kind of facilitative helping relationship is to be established between the body-worker and the patient, then it is vitally important that some emotional contact exist between the two. The body-worker must show that he/she is ready to make contact with the emotional life of the patient. This brings up a range of possibilities. For example, emotional distance may interfere with this type of contact. We recall a conversation between body-work professionals that went something like this: "I just find it hard sometimes to make emotional contact with this patient," said Jane.

"What do you mean?" asked Hermione.

40

"You know, to just know what they are feeling - to perhaps let myself even feel what they are feeling," replied Jane.

Hermione looked baffled and aghast. "What would you want to do that for? You just do your job and that's it, right?"

The conversation stopped there.

Sometimes, the personality of the body-worker is such that they have great difficulty making emotional contact, or even understanding the very concept. This could result from personality features of the body-worker or from her understanding of the nature of the task or dynamics of the process of the body-work. It is our belief that emotional contact is a vital ingredient, a catalyst of the healing process for many patients.

Sometimes patients may have issues with emotional contact. Certain patients may paradoxically need emotional contact, but at the same time be overwhelmed by it when they get it. Sometimes body-workers (or any professional for that matter) will notice that, after they have had a particulary meaningful or emotionally charged session with a client, often one involving a breakthrough, the client misses the next session or perhaps does not show up for a while. It is almost as if the emotional contact with self and the others was too much.

Sometimes difficulties with emotional contact can be manifested in complex ways involving more subtle forms of interpersonal pressure. For example, some patients will act in very "entitled" ways, treating the body-worker as if they are their own servant, acting as if the worker is to respond to their every beck and call, changing appointments, showing up late, expecting special treatment. These behaviors, often combined with less easily observed issues involving tone of voice and gesture, can often evoke in the practitioner feelings of rage and a wish to not be close to the patient. Sometimes this dynamic can be understood as an elaborate technique to reduce contact between the patient and the would-be helper. Frequently, this scenario can be understood as a transference/ countertransference, re-enactment of a mother-child relationship existing in the patient's early history.

If we refer to sections in this book on psychological type (Chapter 12), we can see that certain psychological types will be more prone to making emotional contact of the type being discussed here. For example, extrovert feeling types (especially if there is sufficient development of introversion and introspection) will be prone to establishing emotional contact with others, while introvert thinking types may have some work to do on themselves to increase their emotional availability to others.

Emotional contact is thus a potentially important curative factor in body-work, just as it is in psychological counseling. Empathy is one of the key ingredients to the creation of unconditional positive regard, cited by Rogers (1961) and is vital to the creation of the sense of psychological safety, which Herman (1992) argues is a vital component of the working-through process of trauma. We will discuss the topic of providing a health-promoting psychological surround in Section V, Chapters 16 and 17.

The Music of Touch:

Ashley Montagu in his book entitled "Touch, the Human Significance of the Skin" (1986) gives example after example of how vital touch is to human beings, not just in their sense of well being, but also in their development. The skin is how we communicate with others and a vital way in which we find out about the world around us. Body-workers touch their patients and in that touch they communicate an enormous amount. They not only find out about their patients, about their tensions, their pain and even about their lives, they also communicate to their patients in the way that they touch them. The touch is of course governed by the precepts and rules of technique, but we all know that the same piece of music can sound very different depending on who is playing it, on the touch of the player. Similarly, several massage therapists or naprapaths may all be performing the same technique but the messages they are communicating with their touch, messages that the patient is picking up on, sometimes consciously, sometimes unconsciously, might all be very different. One therapist may be touching very briskly, perhaps brusquely and their patient feels uncared for, perhaps as though they are being dismissed or kept at a distance. The next body-worker is touching very gently, so gently, in fact that the patient feels as though the body worker is afraid of them, is afraid of making contact. The patient perhaps starts to get anxious. The last body-worker may be touching very warmly and firmly, but the patient feels that the touch is too lingering and they perhaps start to feel anxious about the closeness of the therapist. Clearly the possibilities are endless.

Touch is one of the first languages we use to communicate with others. It is through the touch of our early caretakers that we learn about emotions and caring. Manfred Clynes in his fascinating book "Sentics" (1989)has shown that the basic emotions (love, anger, hate, sex, grief, reverence, joy) each have a basic "shape" a basic contour of stimulation and that the human brain seems to be pre-programmed to recognize these in multiple modalities. For example the sharp acceleration and deceleration of anger can be recognized whether it is sonic, visual or kinesthetic, whether a voice is raised sharply and quickly, whether a light flashes on and off quickly, or whether a gesture is sharp and fast. We "know" without even needing words that there is cause for alarm, something is distressed, there is anger, perhaps danger. I would argue that the body-worker, in touching a patient, is rather analogous to a mother communicating to an infant, or the touch of a concert pianist on the keyboard that communicates the essential "feel" of the musical passage. Each of these, in their roles will communicate volumes about feeling and intention through the way they touch either their baby or the keys of the piano. Similarly, if we are angry, or afraid, or joyous, these emotions will be communicated to others and rapidly (and usually quite accurately) picked up by those we are working with. This is part of who we are and it also will become part of the countertransference. For better or for worse, it will have profound impacts on the outcomes of treatments. It behooves us then to become aware of this musical language that we are using to communicate with our patients, this language that is communicated through our tone of voice, our gestures and vitally through the very manner in which we touch and manipulate our patients.

In addition, Clynes' theory helps solve the problem as to why humans have music. Music is a means of communicating these fundamental and precise emotional contours. This communication in a species as social as is ours is vital for survival. Music provides a means of sharpening our "emotion recognition and communication" skills.

On the diagram below we have sketched the basic form of Clyne's Sentic shapes, the shapes of the basic emotions he was able to identify across cultures using his "sentographic transducer." His version and his study are *far* more precise than that which we are illustrating here, but the basic form is similar. (We highly recommend you investigate his research further.)

Diagram 1: Approximations of Clyne's Sentic Shapes

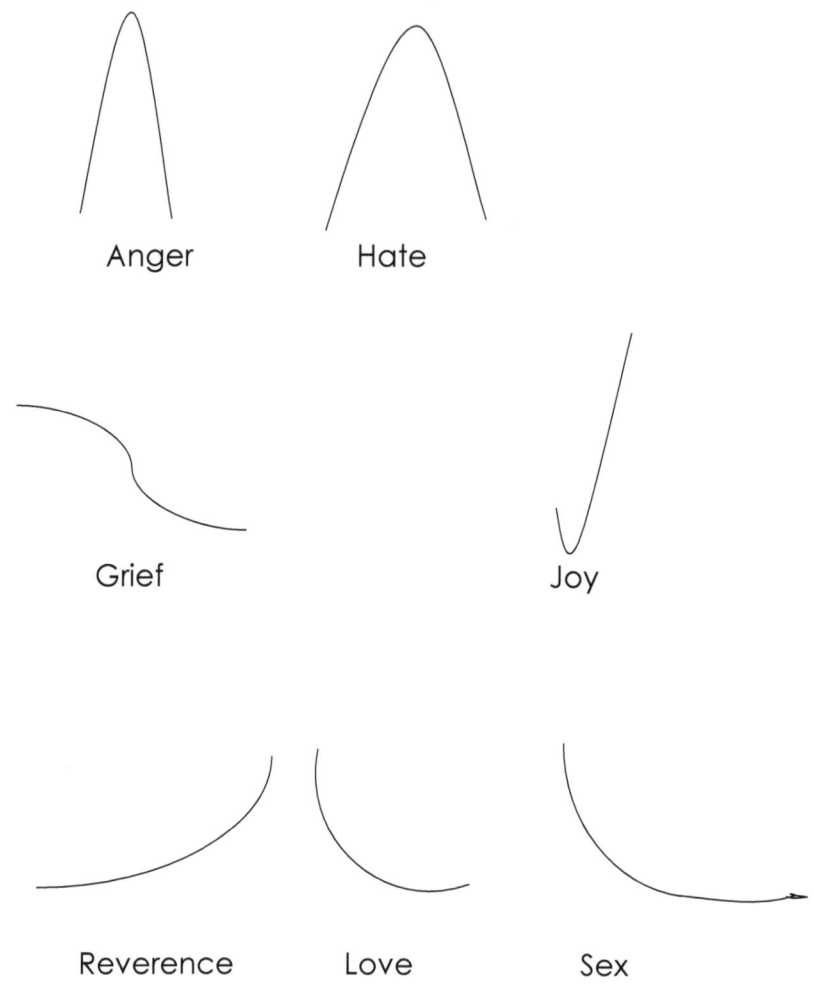

Anger   Hate

Grief   Joy

Reverence   Love   Sex

Each of the shapes captures the essential form of the basic feeling. Imagine that time is running from left to right across the page. Thus, anger is a feeling that involves a sudden onset of stimulation and an equally rapid reduction. It has a jagged shape, like the jagged shapes you see in Picasso's "Guernica," or the sharp jagged sounds of angry music, like heavy metal rock. When people are angry, their voices have a jagged shape and their gestures are sharp-edged. The "shape," the "contour" of the emotion is transferable across all the sensory modalities, and Clynes demonstrates that our reading of the emotion is extremely accurate. If the shape is changed by only a few milliseconds, people soon start to recognize it as another emotion. It is as if our emotion-recognizing device in our brains can be extremely accurate. We have this experience sometimes when we are listening to a piece of music being done by a different performer. For example sometimes the first movement of Mozart's 40th symphony can sound full of foreboding, while another performer makes it sound as if it is to do with longing. What Clynes would argue, I think, is that the shape of the notes is communicating a slightly different amalgam of emotions.

When we apply this to body-work, we can see that the way in which a client is touched or spoken to or communicated to with body language will communicate volumes in comparison to the few sentences that might actually be uttered. If a practitioner is angry, either that day or on a fairly continuous basis, it will be communicated without words through these Sentic forms. Similarly, if the practitioner has a deeply reverential attitude towards the body and his/her work, this too will be communicated through the Sentic forms. Of course, much of what has been covered before will determine what clients prefer and what personal style the body-worker brings to his/her work. The areas of transference and countertransference that were covered earlier will be largely "negotiated" through this mostly unconscious means of communication. It is this type of process that leads us to say things like, "I am not sure why, but I am not comfortable with this person. I cannot put it into words," or "I just get the feeling that he or she really cares about me, like they really respect me," or "I do not know why, but I always feel down after I spend some time with them," or "What is it about that person? They always just cheer me up!" The answer is, of course, that in their process, their tones of voice, their movements and their gestures, there is a dance, a song, and a sculpture, that has to do with the positive emotions.

CHAPTER 4
Classic Body Energy Flows

Diagram 2: Bodily Energy Flows

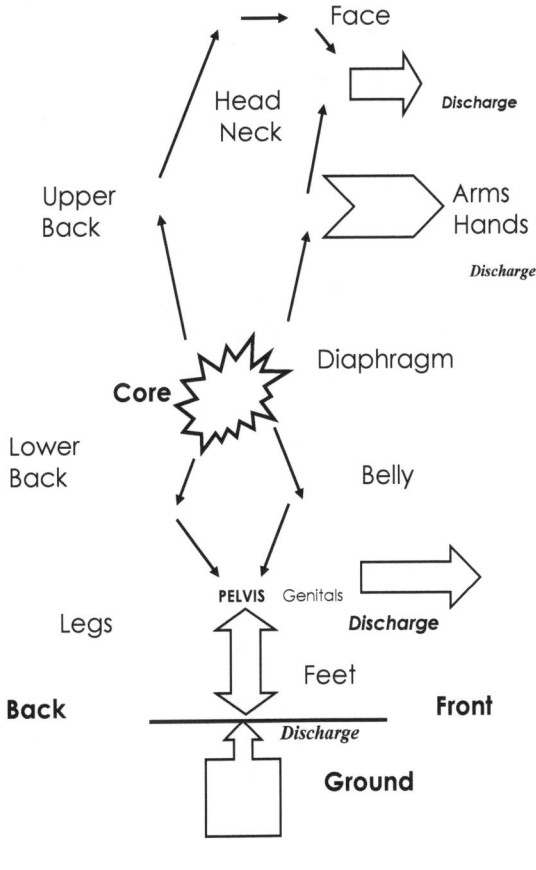

The diagram above shows in very simplified and schematic form the flows of energy through the body hypothesized by Reich and Lowen. We have also added a couple of ideas. For a much fuller exposition of this theory, we highly recommend you visit and study the original works of Reich and Lowen. Your efforts will be amply rewarded. Please bear in mind that this is our interpretation of their work, not necessarily an accurate representation of their thoughts. It also is a clinical theory, which means these ideas have not been proven by traditional scientific means. What they do have going for them, however, is that in our experience they have a terrific amount of clinical utility. Again and again, these ideas help us understand clients and offer assistance to them. It may be that time will refute many of these ideas, but we do believe that many will be shown to have traditional scientific, as well as, clinical validity.

Let us follow the flow of energy through the body, beginning with the core. As we see, energy radiates from the core (approximately the heart-diaphragm/solar plexus region). Energy streams from this central zone up and down the front and back of the body. Each of these four pathways has a distinct and important emotional meaning.

Up the chest, neck to the chin and mouth: This pathway carries the soft, tender, heartfelt feelings—feelings of longing and of melting in love. Often when people feel these feelings they will touch this area of the body as if to emphasize that they are having a heartfelt moment. Tender passages of music capture these emotions and touch this area of the body.

Down the belly and to the genitals: This pathway is associated with the melting feelings of sexuality. It is associated with the tender side of love and sex when we melt into our loved one and lose ourselves in sexual merger.

Up the back, over the head and out the eye teeth: This pathway has to do with aggression, the kind of aggression we see in an animal when it raises its hackles, when its fur rises along its upper spine and when it bares its teeth. Often the eyes will glint and glitter when this energy pathway is activated. Often the energy passes through the shoulder girdle down the arms and into the hands.

Down the lower back, into the buttocks, around and through the pelvis and out the genitals: This pathway has to do with the assertive component of sexuality, the robust, willful reaching out for increased sexual pleasure, for increased depth and extent of sexual pleasurable contact with the other.

This model is fully developed in the work of Reich and Lowen and it is extremely complex. A few examples, however, can serve to illustrate how this model might be applied to some quite common cases.

Trauma will interrupt the flows of these energies, since trauma will cause chronic muscle tensions that will not allow the streaming through of the energy. Thus someone who has had their heart broken, especially in early childhood, will perhaps manifest deep tensions in their chest muscles, their pectorals and intercostals. Perhaps this will radiate into a jutting set jaw and even a tight-lipped, set mouth that almost seems to say, "Never again, will I let my heart get the better of me, and never again will I be hurt like that. I will keep the soft, heartfelt feelings under control."

An individual who grew up with very strict sexual prohibitions and consequent anxieties about their own sexual feelings may develop chronic muscle tensions in both of the downward flowing streams of energy and this might show in tight abdominal muscles, constricted lower back muscles and tensions in the muscles deep in the pelvis.

Individuals who grew up in environments that did not support, or actively undermined, their assertive reaching out for what they wanted, or their pushing themselves off from others (their individuation) may have tense muscles in the shoulder girdle and relatively little energy flowing into their arms and hands.

The diagram hypothesizes that energy is discharged through several channels in the body; through the face and mouth, through the arms, through the genitals and down into the ground through the legs. Chronic muscle tension from trauma can result in energy being dammed up in the body instead of discharging through these channels. This energy becomes stagnant and then toxic, causing both physical and emotional problems. Much body-work aims at opening up these pathways and getting the flow reinstated. What is apparent here, however, is that if we employ this model, these reinstatements of flow will also result in deep changes in the attitudes and behavior of the person. There is a deep isomorphism between body and behavior. Following the work of Reich and Lowen, we believe that a good psychotherapist knows that if their work with a client has been effective, there will be a significant change in the client's body or the attitude the client has to their body. We believe that in parallel form, a course of body-work can be deemed successful if it has resulted in a change in the client's behavior. These behavioral changes may be radical or small. They may involve a change in career or they may involve simply taking up a new hobby or exercise regimen. Many times these "small" changes can carry deep meaning for people. In reclaiming a part of their body that was previously cut off, they have also reclaimed a piece of themselves from which they were previously estranged. For example, Tim, a client who had difficulty standing up for himself took up, as therapy proceeded, bicycle riding. This was associated with him taking stands on things in his life and becoming more assertive.

For example, if a person has body-work that does "open up their chest" it may well be that they start to feel things in a more heartfelt way. Perhaps they and their friends and family are ready for this change. Perhaps they are not. A caring professional can be ready to help if they are equipped with awarenesses like the ones we are proposing here. Similar arguments will apply to all of the simple examples given above. As a result of working on the belly, lower back and pelvic muscles, a client may become aware of sexual feelings and issues they were previously unaware of. Again, this will obviously have repercussions in their personal life.

A patient who comes to a body-worker to release deep chronic tensions in his shoulder girdle, upper back, neck and scalp, may suddenly find he/she is asserting him/herself in unexpected ways at home and at work. He/she may find this exhilarating, but equally, he/she may be afraid, even unwilling to pursue further treatment because unconsciously (perhaps even consciously) he/she knows that it was the treatment that unlocked these physical and emotional flows.

In studying the diagram above of classic bodily energy flows, we see that there are several arrows that indicate pathways of discharge. Various theories and approaches to body-work hypothesize different pathways and avenues of energy discharge. Here we will examine just a few.

Wilhelm Reich argued that the main (perhaps the only) avenue for energy discharge in the body was that of of sexual discharge. More recent thinkers, including Lowen have argued that there are other pathways. It seems intuitively correct that human beings discharge energy through their sexuality. We build up sexual excitement and feel relaxed and often sleepy after an orgasm. This is a typical human experience. This pattern of discharge may relate to body-workers in several ways. For example, even simple body-work can increase the available energy in an individual. Often the immediate effect of, say, a massage is deep sleepiness and relaxation, but following this there could be a rebound and the individual feels more energized. If he/she does not have avenues for discharging this energy, other problems could emerge. Sometimes these might be psychological, such as irritation or anxiety. Sometimes they may show in the person having an increased libido or sexuality. Now, many people may welcome this, but for some personalities and for some individuals from different cultures, this may be quite problematic. Not all individuals nor do all cultures welcome sexuality as a positive life force. Body- workers should be aware of these possibilities.

Lowen argues that bioenergy can be discharged through many avenues in the body. He particularly emphasizes the importance of discharging energy through the legs and into the ground. Following his reasoning, it would follow that when body-work results in a larger amount of available energy in the person, the client should be facilitated in finding ways of discharging that energy in satisfying, life-enhancing ways that promote further well being. For example, walking, cycling, soccer, jogging, Tai Chi, power yoga, swimming, aerobics are all ways of keeping the energy flowing through the organism, and keeping the life force fresh, preventing stagnation of energy. Clearly, body-workers should be aware of the precepts of exercise physiology, kinesiology, as well as these factors under current consideration to help patients in the most appropriate manner.

Energy can also be discharged through the arms and hands and through the voice. Thus when patients, energized by body-work, express an interest in singing, yodeling, guitar, harp, weeding, knitting and so on, these should be regarded as natural outflows of the increased availability of energy to the person. In many ways, they are to be the expected results of successful body-work. Of course, many of these activities are extremely social and this social interaction will often have powerful positive effects on the person's body, amplifying the initial positive effects of the body work. The body-worker, when viewed from this perspective, becomes a potentially radically effective agent of holistic change in the patient's life. He/she is not just working with the patient's body, but with his/her whole biopsychosocial and spiritual organism. With this radical potency, of course, comes a heightened sense of responsibility and care.

Classic Holding Zones in the Body

The work of Reich and Lowen alert us to the fact that there are classic bodily blocking zones, areas of muscular tension, that are extremely common and that often carry similar emotional meanings for their sufferers. Here we will take a very quick tour of these bodily holding zones, recalling that this is but a swift summary and that the reader is strongly recommended to visit the original authors for more complex and detailed input.

The ring from the eyes to the rear base of the skull: Reich argued that bodily holding zones arranged themselves in rings like belts around the body. A very basic ring runs in a circle through the eyes and to the junction of the hard and soft tissue at the base of the rear skull. This ring of tension often holds deep anxieties. (Remember, the theory is that the closer we are to the head, the earlier the developmental impasse). Therefore clinicians working with this area may encounter deep feelings, often of terror, or of lack of support, that clients will find very hard to put into words. Since this blocking zone involves the eyes, it sometimes is involved when people have seen things that traumatized them in some way. Again this blockage can also serve to block the assertive energies that radiate and flow up and over the back of the head and into the face.

Consonant with the theory that development proceeds from the top of the head downward towards our legs, is the observation that the muscles that control the eyes are among the very first to be organized and controlled in the development of the human being. We notice this when we observe infants rise to the challenge of tracking interesting objects through space. The psychologist Jean Piaget (1976) refers to this skill as an essential precursor of the development of "object constancy," the capacity to understand that objects continue to exist, even when we do not directly perceive them. The eyes are extremely important to human beings. We are very visually oriented; large areas of our brains are devoted to vision. In addition, traumatic experiences are often registered in visual form and involve the muscles that move the eyeball. Thus body workers can routinely expect that any exercise that involves the movement of the eyes will potentially engage memories in some form or another of traumatic experiences. (This insight, which owes its origins to Reich and his co-workers, is used to some extent by modern therapists who use the eye movement therapy EMDR (Shapiro and Forrest, 1998)).

The Jaw: Many of the people who did body-work with Wilhelm Reich remarked that he worked intensively with the jaw and that he was able to move his jaw freely and relaxedly, without resistance with his fingers. The jaw is a key zone of tension and of "holding" in the body. Furthermore, tensions in the jaw radiate and involve other areas of the body. A tightly locked jaw can often be associated with tension in the small muscles around the larynx and the neck.

If we examine the diagram of flows of bodily energy, we can easily see that tension in the jaw will block energy flowing from the heart to the mouth. Sometimes it is as if the person is gritting their teeth, saying, "No, I will never speak my heart again!" When the often-painful muscular tensions locked up in the muscles in the jaw are touched, there can be an association with the many complex and deep emotions related to the heart-mouth connection. Often times the sadness and rage at having one's heart broken can be touched upon. Sometimes the fear of taking the risk of speaking one's true feelings can emerge.

Reich and Lowen believed that there was a functional relatedness between the jaw and the pelvis, such that if there was a locking of the jaw, then there could be a similar lack of flexibility in the pelvis. This would have a multiplicity of results: sexual frustrations, difficulties in making emotional contact and, of course, all the pains and aches, especially in the lower back, associated with structural rigidity.

If Reich and Lowen were on the right track here, body-workers palpating either the jaw or the areas in the pelvic region can expect to frequently encounter not only physical but also emotional sensitivities of the rawest and most important kind.

The Neck: The neck has sometimes been referred to by poets as "the narrows" the slim part of the body that connects the heart to the head. In this metaphor we can see that if an individual carries tensions in this area, it may well have to do with the relationship of those two parts of the body and the functions they symbolize. Is this person ruled more by his/her heart than his/her head? Is she afraid her heart will run away with her? Is she afraid she might lose her head? Do the heart and the head bicker or do they co-operate with one another?

We have also encountered quite a surprisingly high number of people who are extremely sensitive to being touched in the neck area because they have been assaulted and held, often to the point of strangulation, in that zone.

Many people carry these anxieties and it seems not totally unreasonable to anticipate that these self same concerns are sometimes carried in the body. As a naprapath, chiropractor, massage therapist or any other body-worker delves into this region of the body, they perhaps should not be surprised when they encounter such concerns in their patient or client. As with each of these areas, we are not even hoping to provide a complete overview of the multitudinous possibilities for mind-body connection in each area of the body. All we are attempting to do is alert the practitioner to some of the possibilities and to stimulate curiosity and interest in this often overlooked but important domain.

The Shoulder Girdle: This region is a step away from the very vulnerable area of the head and its connections to the very earliest stages of emotional development. However, it is a region that can still be very highly charged with feelings and experiences from the past. The shoulders are multi-functional. They engage the arms that reach out to make contact and to express ourselves. We discharge energy through our arms and hands. We make contact through our arms and hands. We also use the shoulders self-protectively, to brace ourselves against an emotional or physical shock, and to activate the arms in pushing away something we do not want in our space or in our face. The shoulders stand metaphorically for robustness, assertion, responsibility, autonomy, self-direction, and self-control. These issues typically manifest themselves vigorously in toddlers, often in very powerful ways as they experiment actively with the world around them, testing it and their limits.

A most cursory observation of humanity informs us that these issues are found with a very high degree of frequency. Some individuals have frozen their shoulder girdle in a chronic position of upward self inflation, as if to tell the world, "Don't even think of messing with me!" Others have very undercharged shoulders and arms, as if to say, "Do not worry. I will not assert myself and grab!" Yet others may be locked into a permanent posture of self-protection, with frozen, braced shoulders, as if to say, "I am ready for the next blow."

Another frequent pattern is found in the person who has perhaps had to "carry the world on their shoulders," often with very little help. He may have been called upon to take up early and extra responsibilities in his family, owing to the absence of an effective parental figure. Sometimes this person will have a hunched posture and a very well developed pad of muscle on his upper back.

Sometimes, one can see a person who has had to "rise above the situation," and this might show in a significant upward displacement of energy and mass in his/her body. His shoulders become broad and wide, while his legs are less well developed. The raising of the shoulders seems to serve the purpose of demonstrating to him/herself and the world that he is strong and in control.

All these and many more issues can be found in the tight contractions and constrictions of the shoulders. We must also recall that, since the body is a functional unit, these tensions will reverberate throughout the entire body system. For example, tight rigid shoulders will affect the weight-bearing function of the spine, pelvis, knees, right down to the arches in the feet. Again, body-workers, after reading these paragraphs, will perhaps not be surprised the next time they are working with a client's shoulders and the client resists the work with a groan not only of pain, but also of anxiety as age-old postures that have meant so much for so long are called metaphorically into question by the palpation of the involved muscles.

The Chest: As with all the other areas of the body, armoring in the chest can serve many functions. It is also of vital significance because the chest is associated with such important functions as the lungs and the heart. It is also our core, it helps stabilize and energize most of the other movements in the body.

Sometimes the chest is rigidified to protect the heart. The intercostal muscles, the muscles between the ribs, sometimes seem to be tightened as if this will protect one from being hurt again and of ever having to suffer again the pain and disappointment of having his heart broken.

Sometimes the chest is hyperinflated, as if to protrude into the world and to dominate it, perhaps in compensation for a deeper sense of helplessness and insignificance. Then again, the reverse situation might obtain, where an individual deflates and flattens his chest so as not to appear as a threat and thus ward off competition from others.

The chest is also a means of making contact with others. Chest-to-chest contact is very important and can be very bonding and comforting to many primates. Thus, we can see in the chest attitudes of readiness to make contact or of an avoidance or mistrust of contact.

The chest is also involved in breathing, the seat of our aliveness and energy. An immobile chest and shallow breathing is often associated with depression or in attempts to block feelings that might emerge into awareness should the person breathe more deeply and thus become more energized.

Naprapaths and all body-workers will almost always involve work directly or indirectly with the chest, this area that is the seat of so many emotional responses and attitudes toward life and others. In so doing, they are potentially opening up long-standing issues in their patients.

The Abdomen/Lower Back Girdle: When we examine the diagram at the beginning of this section, we see that energy passes from the core, down the belly, into the genitals and legs, and from the core, down the lower back, through the pelvis, into the genitals, and down the legs into the ground. Lowen argues that the energy flowing down the front, down the belly, is associated with the softer, melting feelings involved in the sexual encounter, while the energy flowing down the lower back has to do with the more assertive aspects of sexuality. Ideally, these two forms of energy are integrated so that there is the joy of melting into the other in sexuality, combined with the necessary assertion to bridge the gap to the other. Rene Spitz, a French psychiatrist, has a useful analogy of assertion acting as a "carrier wave" for the feelings of tenderness and that metaphor seems to fit well here. It is all very well to love and feel tender, but it is also a good thing to have enough "oomph" to get that message of tenderness across to the other person.

People frequently have issues in these areas, namely the areas of melting tenderness and assertion which, taken together, would come across as a warm assertion or vigorous loving. Sometimes we can see a fear on one side or another of the equation. Someone may be very anxious about giving in to the feelings of tenderness in sexuality and love and this may show in an extremely rigid belly. A retracted pelvis brought on by tightness in the muscles of the lower back may indicate an unconscious anxious attitude regarding assertiveness in sexuality or an anxiety regarding contact with the other.

As a result of these types of tensions, the pelvis can be locked in a tilted position that places undue strain on the spine and hip joints and that radiates throughout the body. These types of tensions are often found in people who have been sexually abused. As we have argued many times before in this book, when a body-worker attempts to unfreeze and mobilize this zone, he or she is, if we follow these arguments, stepping into an area of emotions and ideas that, although they may be largely unconscious, are, nevertheless, extremely highly charged.

The Pelvic Region: Armoring in the pelvic region, the buttocks, hips and into the pelvic floor are quite clearly related to sexuality. As such, this area is usually very prone to a high charge of energy and suffused with layers of extra meaning. One can imagine all of the "scripting" one has received in one's life regarding sexuality, all the messages and all the experiences, both positive and negative, as being nested, perhaps knotted up in this region of the body. The lucky individual will be relatively free of deep tensions in this area, while many will carry deep sensitivities and anxieties here.

The possibilities are legion, so just a few examples will provide some sketching out of the territory. For example, an individual may have grown up in a very sexually restrictive environment and learned to suppress his/her sexual impulses through a tensioning of many of the muscles in this region. Consequently, the body-worker will encounter pain and anxiety when engaging these muscles, tendons and ligaments. Since the pelvis is such a central part of the body, it is quite likely that the body-worker will engage these zones even though he/she is working with a section of the body that seems far away from the pelvis.

The tissue in the buttocks, in bioenergetic theory, is claimed to be a reservoir of sexual energy, storing up the charge somewhat like a capacitor before the discharge during orgasm. The gluteal muscles are involved in this process. Thus when body-workers are engaging these muscles, they are potentially altering the charge/discharge balance in the individual's sexuality. Some individuals will experience this with considerable discomfort and anxiety.

The hip flexors are involved in the free rotation of the pelvis atop the legs. This free rotation is involved in the free expression of sexuality. Body-workers will not infrequently be called upon to work on the hip flexors and the related muscles that enable the free rotation of the pelvis. In individuals with "life scripts" that prohibit the full expression of their sexuality, this will be a process complicated not only by bodily considerations, but also by the psychological and emotional impacts.

SECTION II
Biopsychosocial Development Challenges and the Body

We have already argued that traumatic experiences are "stored" in the body in different regions. Trauma will also tend to lock a person, physically, socially and psychologically at a given developmental stage. For example, we have already argued that earlier trauma will perhaps be "locked into" areas closer to the head than issues that develop later in childhood. If the individual is working on issues of dependence/independence, trust/mistrust at such early stages of life then a fixation, or a complex will occur around these issues. These issues will manifest in all realms of the person's biopsychosocial being. Perhaps, by examining several developmental theories, we can arrive at a more detailed and thus more useful view.

CHAPTER 5

Erik Erikson: The Life Cycle and the Body

Erikson's eight stages of psychosocial development (1963) are widely known. As can be seen on Table 1, each stage consists of a focal conflict between two opposites—trust/mistrust; autonomy/shame and doubt, and so on. Each stage builds on the previous stage, and, if successfully negotiated, results in a corresponding psychological strength, or virtue. If, for some reason, the task of integrating the opposites into some functional synthesis is not accomplished, then the work of the succeeding stages becomes that much more difficult and a distortion corresponding to the stage is created. For example, the individual who is unable to form a sufficiently durable sense of trust is liable to form the distortion of "idolism" and will have a pronounced tendency to worship others or themselves as if still seeking that perfect, trustworthy person. Each stage rests upon the repeated performance of a "ritualization," an activity that helps in the accomplishment of the integrative task of a given stage. Readers can find a more detailed account of Erikson's theory in Chapter 2 of "Family Systems Activity Book" (Hazell, 2006).

Further, when we turn to the original source (Erikson 1963), we see that Erikson's theory is radically embodied. By this we mean that each stage, for Erikson, is not only psychosocial, it is also physical. Each stage involves bodily modalities, regions and processes that he takes pains to describe.

This has consequences for our present purpose. It implies that the resolution of each psychosocial stage will have correspondences in bodily processes—correspondences of which the body-worker may need to be aware. Not only will the client's resolution of the psychosocial stages show up in his personal style and how he interacts in treatment, they will also manifest in the patient's physical style.

Table 1 gives a quick summary of some of the correspondences between Erikson's stages and bodily modalities that are involved in each stage. The ages are approximate and alter over time and place.

Table 1 :   Correspondences between Erikson's Stages and Bodily Modalities

STAGE	BODILY MODALITIES
Trust – Mistrust(0-1yr)	Taking in, absorbing, relaxing, being held.
Autonomy – Shame/Doubt(2-3yrs)	Holding on, letting go, controlling, willing, directing. Muscular control. Locomotion. Affirming/negating.
Initiative – Guilt(3-5yrs)	Projecting into space, enclosing. Moving around, adventuring, playing.
Industry – Inferiority(5-12yrs)	Expanding with competent pride. Contracting with feelings of inferiority. Learning.
Identity – Identity Confusion(12-25yrs)	Coherence and continuity of body image vs. fragmentation of body image. Positive and negative feelings about the body.
Intimacy – Isolation(20-40yrs)	Melting into the other, becoming as one vs. maintaining one's own physical boundaries. Give and take.
Generativity – Stagnation(40-old age)	Caring for the bodies of others now and in the future versus ceasing to grow, sponsor, coach, train and mentor—giving up on the body.

Ego Integrity – *Despair(Advanced old age to* *death)*	Coping with bodily decline and disintegration. Integration of bodily identity.

While we are working on these developmental challenges all the time, during critical eras of life, certain conflicts emerge into prominence. Sometimes, unfortunate circumstances prevent the complete resolution of certain developmental issues. This leads to predictable psycho-social patterns of behavior. In addition it leads to typical patterns, sometimes problematic, in bodily modalities.

These developmental issues may manifest in the course of body-work. Let us walk through each of the eight stages of Erikson's theory and give an example or two of how issues emanating from each stage may show up in the process of working with the body.

Trust – Mistrust

A patient who has issues regarding trust and mistrust may have difficulties absorbing physical and psychological nourishment, holding on to such a nutrient and growing from it. Such absorption involves trust. Such a patient may find it hard to relax on the table and may not be able to hold on to the good aspects of treatment for long or to even let the goodness soak in. Such an attitude can prove frustrating to the clinician who wishes to help and see results. Such frustration can be eased, however, if the deeper understanding being proposed here, namely that the difficulties arise from issues in early childhood in establishing a trusting relationship, is entertained.

On the other hand, a patient who perhaps never received enough love and attention during this crucial early stage of life may be very greedy, as if no amount of care and attention is enough. They may act in a very entitled fashion, asking for special favors, extra time, preferential treatment and, in addition, not acknowledging it when it is given.

Issues related to trust and mistrust can also be seen in the body language of patients. For example, patients having trust and mistrust issues may become anxious as they lie down on the treatment table, or a look of fear may show in their eyes as they become more vulnerable.

Certain clients can only be touched, for example, in well-armored areas of their body, their back, for instance.

With clients who manifest these kinds of issues the therapist can take a gradualist approach to gaining trust. Perhaps even establishing an alliance with the patient which is aimed at helping the patient to relax and absorb the benefits of treatment. Sometimes patients who have trust issues will sabotage the treatment in various ways. The self-sabotage sometimes seems aimed at undermining the positive experiences coming from treatment before they go too far, before there is too much of a chance of a big letdown. This self-sabotage can take many forms: calling up an unpleasant or difficult person right after treatment, doing activities that undermine progress, refusing to follow through on recommendations regarding, say, nutrition and exercise. The clinician will perhaps help the client by tactfully offering this interpretation when the timing seems right.

Autonomy – Shame/Doubt

Many parts of the body and bodily movements have to do with expressions of autonomy, shame, self doubt and will. The very act of standing on our own two feet or of walking implies our own capacity for self control or self direction. A set jaw can express our willfulness. Sagging shoulders, a drooping head or a tilted pelvis, as if we have our tail tucked between our legs, can all be expressions of shame.

Clearly when a body-worker works on these areas of the body, it is likely that such issues will surface, perhaps in the form of feelings that emerge in the course of treatment or in ways that undermine the course of treatment. For example, the body-worker may assign exercises that attempt to overcome a forward head carriage, or that involve loosening the pelvis or simply walking. Each of these exercises may stimulate in the patient an anxiety related to past negative experiences around expressions of their autonomy.

One might also encounter patients who have difficulties in softening their will sufficiently to allow themselves to be influenced by the doctor or body worker. Such individuals may show up to treatment but only allow themselves to be affected by treatment surreptitiously and may even vow that the treatment has not affected them much, when it has in fact had quite a dramatic effect upon them.

Case Example: Trust and Body-work. *Brett showed up at Anita's*

Naprapathic office suffering from pain and reduced mobility in his right arm. Anita diagnosed his situation as resulting from deep tensions in and around his shoulder and she started to palpate the muscles and ligaments around the gleno-humoral process. At first, things proceeded well, but after a while she felt Brett resisting her pressure. She paused and pointed this out, adding that if he trusted her and "let her in" it might hurt temporarily, but that it would ultimately be to his benefit, that his pain would be relieved and his range of motion increase. Brett, following this was able to relax his defense and let Anita work the deeper layers of tissue and, fortunately, did feel better and regain range of motion.

This vignette contains deep and interesting material in its apparent simplicity. Key among its contents is the concept of trust. The treatment could only progress if Brett was able to _trust_ Anita. In part this trust will rest on his perception of her competence, along with how she presents herself and her actual competence. In part it also depends on his _transference_ on to Anita, the extent to which he has been able to trust other influential persons in his life, such as his parents, and the extent to which he transfers these feelings and expectations onto Anita, his doctor.

In this case vignette Anita is able to explicitly ask for the trust, gain it and effectively follow through with the treatment. Brett was also able to marshal his trust, transfer it onto Anita and, literally, put himself in her hands.

Initiative vs. Guilt

Initiative has to do with the framing of purposes and carrying them into effect. It builds upon the previous stages yet it adds its own essential ingredients. One of these is the linkage and coordination of parts to achieve an end in the future.

Body-work will frequently involve just such an integration and coordination on a bodily level. When we create an integrated body image that can be directed to a goal, we can more readily exercise our initiative. When we connect our vision to our ideas and then link these to our backbone, legs and hands in a coordinated plan, we are primed to exercise initiative.

Clearly such body-work does precisely this kind of linkage work and this can liberate long dormant initiatives in the client. As these initiatives (to start a business or a family, to make a trip, to take a course) surface, so will a complex of feelings to which the body-worker should be sensitive. If these feelings are not met and understood, the integrative body-work could be stalled.

The case of Brad gives an idea of one way a patient may behave if they have unresolved issues of autonomy and initiative.

Case Example Resistance to Change: *Brad, a 35-year-old man weighed 280 pounds and was five feet eight inches tall. His primary complaint was rib pain at thoracic vertebra twelve, but he complained of a wide array of problems, involving digestion, headaches and diffuse pain.*

The body-worker did her best to reach the problem in the back (which she thought was due to a rotated rib) but it was very difficult to access owing to thick layers of muscle and a hypersensitivity to touch and pressure that she thought was due to build-up of toxins in the body from poor diet and lack of exercise.

The body-worker prescribed a program of exercise and a sequence of treatment sessions. Brad continually missed sessions and did not do any exercises. His condition did not improve and he continued in his complaints. The doctor, who, quite naturally, liked to see her patients improve, became first frustrated then resigned and despondent. The cycle continued.

The case of Brad can be understood by referring to the theories of Mahler (see Chapter 6) and Erikson. Using these theories we would hypothesize that Brad's separation and individuation process had not been completed. The activities the doctor was prescribing were the kind of activity (walking, cycling, etc.) that one finds in more individuated children (that is, children who have successfully separated themselves psychologically from their mothers). Brad resisted these activities because he symbolically did not want to experience himself as a separate individual.

We may also hypothesize that Brad had issues with Erikson's stage of autonomy—shame, doubt. This is evidenced by his shrinking from the activities that would be associated with the expression of will (which is associated with the autonomy-shame/doubt stage). It is as if he would be asserting himself and increasing his autonomy by activating his body in certain ways.

In addition, Brad evinced many of the qualities of what has been called "the help-rejecting complainer." He would recurrently complain and often whine about his condition while at the same time seem to willfully refuse to do the very things that would help him get better.

Slowly the body-worker became aware, through the fog of her frustration and Brad's complaining, that Brad as a little boy had not received sufficient support for his individuality and, as a consequence, had found it hard to separate from his mother. The doctor realized that the treatment might take some time. Brad was not simply "doing exercises," he was involved in a deep-rooted struggle to lay claim to his own body, mobility and volition. Viewed from this perspective, the doctor was able to be more deeply understanding of Brad, more patient and, ultimately, more helpful.

Industry – Inferiority

It is during this stage that the child swells with pride as he/she gains competencies or shrinks in feelings of low self-worth as he/she is made to feel inferior when he/she cannot perform culturally-valued tasks. We come home glowing with pride bearing good quiz results or we skulk and shrink in anguished shame when we fail.

Erikson seems to argue that this motivation toward competence is genetically pre-programmed. As such, it is bound to be powerful. This often overlooked drive can encode its history in the body. Thus, the body-worker should not be surprised if a course of treatment of the body results in the patient getting in touch with deep-seated feelings and ideas about his/her competence. Wilhelm Reich claimed that a sure way to undermine a person's self-confidence was to disrupt his/her sense of connection to his/her body. Body-work will often re-establish connection between the self and the body. In so doing it will re-establish a sense of confidence and competence in the client. The bodywork practitioner might not then be surprised to see a rise in patients' self esteem and the taking on by the patient of new projects and challenges.

Identity vs. Identity Confusion

During the period of adolescence, the psychosocial task involves the realization of a stable identity. This is an intensely bodily process insofar as one's self image is powerfully affected by one's body image. Body-work again can intervene at this level. Clients may, as a result of body-work, alter their body image, and thus their identity. This can be very profound and have far-reaching effects—on career, marriage, religion, hobbies and relationships. Again, given this line of reasoning, the body-worker should not be surprised when the client starts to see him/herself in a new and different way.

Case illustration, Reclaiming the Body: *Cindy, a sensitive and gifted sixteen- year-old girl had recently suffered a date rape and had been recently discharged from an inpatient program at a local hospital. She was still very agitated and suffered from flashbacks and anxiety attacks. The body-worker had to be very careful in the ways in which she contacted the young woman, as so much pain seemed to be stored in her body. After a few sessions passed and some trust had been established, Cindy happened to mention that she used to love horse riding, but had not done any recently. The body-worker took the hint and, half jokingly, wrote out a prescription, "Horse riding PRN". The body-worker felt that Cindy, as an adolescent, was at some risk for forming her identity around the trauma and its sequelae. She also felt that contact with the horse, with her body, with nature and with a past part of herself would be very good for her in the recovery process. Cindy fulfilled the prescription, went riding and came back the following week with tales of happy memories and loving feelings toward the new horse that she had befriended.*

This case also nicely demonstrates the utility of sports, activities and hobbies in regaining contact and energy in parts of the body that might be "thirsty for action".

Intimacy vs. Isolation

Erikson, in "Childhood and Society" (1963), emphasizes that this stage involves the body. In sexual intimacy we bring our body into close contact with another and let ourselves "flow into" the other and become part of them. Erikson argues (and he has been criticized on this) that this capacity rests upon the establishment of a secure identity. The person who is unsure of their identity (and this, in turn, can result from difficulties encountered in any of the previous stages—it is hard to be intimate if one has a surfeit of mistrust, for example) will have problems letting themselves lose themselves in a love relationship.

Body-workers quite probably will work with clients who are in this psychological stage. They may find that as clients work successfully through bodily related issues there are surprising developments in the client's intimate life—in their relational world. For example, a client who learns to trust himself more as a result of body-work may find it easier to trust others. Issues arising from such growth may be brought to the body-worker's attention.

Generativity vs. Stagnation

In this, the stage of middle age, the conflict is between maintaining a creative, productive flexibility in helping one's community and the world versus a rigid, dead concern with the rules alone and showing no caring for others and the future.

Bodily problems and rigidity are very common during this period of life. Body-workers are very likely to encounter people at this stage. Body-work often results in greater flexibility and this bodily aliveness will translate into increased vitality and generativity. In turn, this generativity will feed aliveness and flexibility. Thus, the effective body-worker will perhaps be intervening (albeit unintentionally and indirectly) in the dynamics of this stage, often facilitating generativity.

Ego Integrity vs. Despair

In this stage, the stage of old age, the individual confronts issues of despair coupled with death and disease. In reaction to this there is an attempt, often through studying the wisdom of the ages, to develop a sense of ego integrity, a sense of being "together" in a dignified coherent way.

The body-worker working with this developmental cohort will inevitably confront these complex issues—clients who manifest despair and disgust over their bodies that perhaps seem to be in rebellion, clients asking deep existential questions on the meaning of life, clients developing a deep sense of faith in the ultimate meaningfulness of their lives.

This, the last stage, is clearly, profoundly embodied and the body-worker will implicitly be asked to be a companion to the elder as they struggle with this, the ultimate dialectic.

There is a growing literature on the study of aging. We have found Tobin's work (1988) to be extremely helpful.

Conclusion

We have "walked through" the eight stages of Erikson's developmental theory and examined some of the implications these developmental challenges have for body-workers. The overall suggestion here, as throughout the entire book, is that when we touch and work with the body, we engage ourselves in crucial psychosocial as well as biological processes.

CHAPTER 6
Mahler's Theory of Separation/ Individuation and Working with the Body

Mahler (1975) presents us with a theory of development that asserts that while the physical birth is established at age zero, psychological birth is a much longer process, taking at least the first 2-3 years of life, and, in many ways, extending over the entire life span.

Diagram 3 gives a visual representation of Mahler's scheme. In the first month, the stage of *normal autism,* the baby is seen as being very withdrawn into itself, sleeping much of the time, and basically attempting to maintain physiological homeostasis. It is the "preobjectal" stage, the era of life before we are aware of the sense of self and other. (Daniel Stern and others (2000), by the way, have challenged this and other concepts of Mahler's, stating, for example, that we enter the world primed to form relationships with others.)

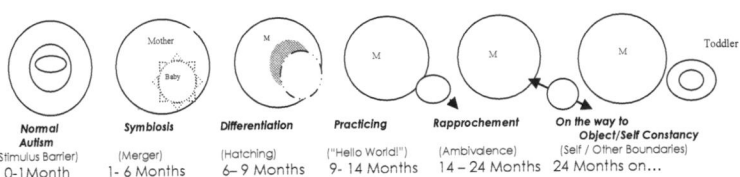

Diagram 3: Schematic of Mahler's Conception of the Separation-Individuation Process

The second stage is that of *symbiosis*, and extends from one to approximately 6 months. During this stage, the baby is in a merged state with its caretaker. There is much mutual gazing, and the infant moulds itself to the mother in what appears to be a state of fusion or oneness.

The next stage of *differentiation* is ushered in as the baby starts to show an interest in that which is other than mother. The baby starts to grasp objects, scan the surrounding world and brace himself using his back muscles. This process is called *hatching*. The baby even develops, during this stage, a certain look in its eyes, the "hatched look", where the baby has a more focused, sharp, curious look in his eyes. Babies in this phase are beginning to be aware of their separateness from their mother. They are very interested in the "other than mother world," other people, earrings, eyeglasses, interesting objects across the room.

By nine or ten months, the baby has become a proto-toddler— able to sit up and scoot around on his own by some form of crawling, able to hold himself erect and cruise from one support to another, and eventually, able to walk. This is called the *practicing subphase*. Here the child shows a great interest in exploring the world, exploring actively, as long as mother is nearby. It is as though the child has a "love affair with the world," buttressed by an internal assumption that his mother is always only a short distance away.

Eventually this over-riding urge to explore is counterbalanced by a need to be in close contact with the mother again, and we see the ambivalence that is the hallmark of the *rapprochement subphase*. During this phase, the toddler seems to want to be apart but also to merge, or at least be in contact with his mother. It is as if his script is, "go away a little closer" or "come here a little further away." At times, the outside world will overwhelm him and he will wish to be picked up by his mother (or caretaker) but then, once picked up, he will want to be set down again only to be picked up again. This stage requires a great deal of patience on the part of the mother. At both this age and the preceding practicing stage, we notice that children will pile things from the outside world in their mother's lap, as if to connect the outside world with their center, their mother.

The rapprochement subphase resolves itself gradually as the child more fully establishes a secure sense of himself as being both a separate person, with his/her own identity, and as having a secure attachment to home base, his/her mother. This security is underpinned by the child having established *affective object constancy*, the capacity to evoke an image in his mind of his mother, and all that she stands for- -warmth, acceptance, hope, support and trust. The mother in previous stages has been a bridge between herself and the outside world. The internalized mother continues to serve this function of linking the child to the outside world.

This, in very brief form, is Mahler's theory. We highly recommend turning to Mahler's (1975) original work. It is a challenging but very worthwhile read. Even though several aspects of his theory have been since challenged (Stern, 2000), many aspects of his work still retain their clinical utility. The next question is, "How does this relate to bodywork?" The answer is, "In very, very many ways." Let us examine a few.

People can get "stuck" to varying extents in each of the subphases, resulting in fairly specific personality traits and reactions to various type of body-work. Let us walk through each subphase and give an example (or two) of how a "fixation" at each stage might manifest itself in body-work. Recall that the developmental process of separation-individuation is lifelong, so we should expect to see change, progression, along the stages beyond those theorized by Mahler even as we work with people, so as long as there is healthful developmental context.

An individual who has significant parts of his personality fixated in the phase of *normal autism*, for example, may be rather unavailable to human emotional contact and may even find contact of this kind unpleasant, or perhaps overstimulating. A body-worker working with an individual with this type of personality should be aware of this and be careful not to overreact when the patient does not seem to respond in what seems to be a contactful way. When persons like this seem to be distant or unconnected, some people can become angry, since they feel rejected and, instead of making themselves available to the patients, they may withdraw or even retaliate.

The *symbiotic* stage is indeed evocative of many different interpersonal patterns. For example, sometimes people have a deep "symbiotic" wish to be understood without words, and they are hurt and upset when this symbiotic fantasy is not realized. Thus, body-work can be at times profoundly evocative of the symbiotic feeling of deep connectedness of self with other, or of the deep frustrations that can occur when the profound wishes are not realized.

The symbiotic era is not always a pleasurable Eden. Some individuals have had very distressed symbiotic stages. They may thus avoid many situations that evoke symbiotic-like feelings or be surprised at negative emotions that arise when they unexpectedly find themselves in a symbiotic situation.

Many bodyworking situations involve the stimulation of symbiotic-like states of mind – one becomes profoundly relaxed and self-other boundaries become fuzzy. For many people this type of regression can be very healthy – a sort of "regression in the service of the ego," but for some it can be quite anxiety producing.

Case Vignette: Mr. P: Rebuilding through a Positive Symbiosis. *Mr P. was a fifty-five year old African American male who came to the clinic complaining of multiple physical aches and pains. He also announced quite clearly that he was unemployed, on disability payments and had been diagnosed with "schizophrenia". His dress was seen by the clinic staff as rather bizarre and he used the neologisms and rituals when he was anxious. Frequently a look of fear would pass through his eyes. His body was tight, thin and stiff, his clothes old and frayed. The body-worker overcame an initial sense of countertransference anxiety and set to work. She very soon noticed some very strong emotional responses, both in herself and in Mr. P. . First, as he lay down on the treatment table, a very soft look came into his eyes and as the sheet was placed over him, the body-worker felt a very strong sense of inclusive protectiveness, "just like he was a little baby". She proceeded with the treatment regimen—stretching, pulling, palpation and pressure and when it was over, Mr. P's body had markedly softened and his eyes were full, soft and liquid. It took him some time to compose himself and the body-worker felt a remarkable sense of tenderness for this strange man whom many of the other staff found odd and even repulsive.*

Mr P. came to sessions religiously and the same intense feelings of connectedness persisted. On several occasions, Mr. P. shared with the body-worker that he loved her. This love, however was not experienced by the body-worker as sexual or threatening. It was a sweet, delicate and tender feeling, like the feelings one has for babies. Mr. P. also shared, on several occasions, that the body-worker had saved his life. The body-worker had the distinct impression that this was not just to do with the relief of pain, which had been considerable, but had more to do with the sense of having one's psychological existence sustained by fusion with an empathic and caring other.

Interestingly, Mr. P's behavior started to change considerably after a few months of treatment. He enrolled in a computer class and started to talk about different topics, topics in the news, his goals for the future. The clinic staff also started to relate to him differently.

The story of Mr. P. can be understood quite effectively if we apply some of the ideas from Mahler's theory. We can see that he swiftly slipped into a positive symbiotic transference state with the body-worker and was able to gain psychological nourishment from this state. This transference/countertransference situation is very close to those described by Harold Searles (1979)in his work with persons diagnosed with schizophrenia. One way of understanding some of the forms of this condition is too see it as a fixation at the symbiotic level. Body-work, with its emphasis on non-verbal relating, is ideally suited to enabling a non-toxic, well bounded, temporary, imaginary symbiotic experience which can provide sufficient emotional capital to strengthen the client's ego such that functionality is enhanced.

These concerns are not the exclusive domain of the patient. Healthcare professionals, body-workers themselves will have varying concerns regarding symbiosis, and their willingness to make emotional contact with their patient or client will be affected by it. Countertransference issues, for example can be very strong in this domain, as the work of Harold Searles (1979), Racker (1968), Winnicott (1965a) and Hirsch (2008) amply illustrate.

The *differentiation subphase* begins around six months of age and is accompanied by some significant physiological changes. The infant now has more control over the trunk muscles and is able to brace himself and to hold himself erect from the waist up. The trunk is thus a "midwife" of the separation process. The infant is now able to arch his back, to no longer mold into the mother's body and to search the world with his gaze. He can scan his mother's face and compare it to other faces. He can now grasp objects and is especially interested in objects that are attached to his mother's body—eyeglasses, earrings, necklaces. The focal distance of his eyes have shifted such that it is easier for him to focus on objects across the room, rather than on objects about nine inches away. All of these make the infant aware of his separation from his mother. He starts to become aware, with varying degrees of sharpness, of this separation. This is a crucial period in the history of the individual. For some this period is a fascinating initial recognition of one's separation and one's individuality. For others this can be a terrifying realization of one's aloneness and isolation. Yet again, some mothers, recognizing that their symbiotic infant is leaving the nest and moving away, feel abandoned and may seek to subvert the infant's separation, perhaps by restricting its movement or facial exploration, perhaps more subtly by becoming depressed or disapproving whenever the infant moves their body in a differentiated way.

Recall that this unfolding is occurring before the arrival of language and that it is a powerfully charged physical experience. The fact that it is very early in life means that it will be a set of learnings deep in the unconscious. It will be a set of learnings, however, that will emerge when the body is subjected to certain experiences—learnings that will perhaps emerge in the course of body-work. Thus, for example, work that helps energize the trunk or neck and increases the motility of these regions, work that facilitates grasping and work that increases proprioception—the sense of one's very own body—may all tap into the "codings" in the patient's unconscious that have to do with the differentiation subphase. Again, for some patients, this may be experienced as a marvelous revelation of their own uniqueness, experienced in an emergent, preverbal way—an inchoate yet moving recognition of one's own wonderful body processes that are uniquely, one's own. On the other hand, the patient's experience may be of a frightening feeling of isolation and abandonment as unconscious codings—memories—of a differentiation subphase which was characterized by experiences of profound aloneness—are activated and re-experienced. In the latter case, of course, forward movement in the treatment could be compromised as the patient seems to have negative responses whenever the trunk, arms or proprioception are activated.

In the *practicing subphase*, at about nine months of age, the child's body undergoes some more significant changes and these lead, again, to significant changes in the soon-to-be-toddler's world and his relationships with others. It is at about this time that the child becomes able in some way or another to move about—he/she starts to crawl, roll, tug, scoot and sometimes even walk around. As he does so he encounters an exciting new world of expansive possibilities. For a few months there is a sort of "love affair with the world," as he temporarily suspends his attachment to his mother and explores the big world and all its possibilities. The child starts to encounter other people, places, and things, and, while often checking back to his mother as a secure base, he will explore them with fascination.

It is not hard to see how the activation of the parts of the body involved in this developmental stage (especially, say, the legs) at a later point in life, perhaps through body-work, may stimulate emotional issues. For this stage, as Mahler amply documents, is not always smooth flowing. Some children may not feel they have a mother who acts as a secure base and thus inhibit their exploratory drives. When they later encounter a therapist who encourages the activation of their legs and free movement in space, these old issues around independence may emerge, sometimes confounding the treatment process if not adequately addressed and if, again, the appropriate support is not given to the patient.

The practicing subphase ends at about 14 months when the *rapprochement subphase* is ushered in. By now, most children are able to walk and move away from their mothers. Also, by now, most children, in the course of their explorations, have had encounters with the outside world that have overwhelmed them, frightened them, or hurt them. Other children may have taken their toys, dogs may have bitten them; they may have gotten lost and scared by strangers. During this stage, the child is not yet secure enough or wise enough in the ways of the world to be fully separate and yet she also wishes to be separate from her mother. She desires the comforting embrace of her mother while also fearing that she may engulf her and compromise her cherished wish for independence. The child in the rapprochement stage is thus caught in the horns of a dilemma. On the one hand they want to be picked up and comforted. On the other hand they want to be left alone. On the one hand they wish to be free and independent; on the other, they dread being abandoned.

Again, we can see how these wishes and fears can easily be seen in adults as they approach and avoid others; as they oscillate from closeness to distance, seemingly never finding a comfortable position in relation to the other. Such ambivalence can also be quite easily seen, we believe in the behavior of many patients in body work. At first they may seem eager for a treatment that will "set them free," only to cease treatment just when it seems to be succeeding. Or, they may request some deep understanding from the therapist, only to recoil when in fact it is forthcoming. Mothers with toddlers of this age are called upon to display great patience. Perhaps the same can be said of professionals who are working with patients with issues emanating from this era. For issues there can be; not all mothers can make themselves patiently available and withstand the intense flood of emotions from the entire spectrum that can accompany this passionate and conflicted stage of childhood.

Aspects of the separation/individuation process may be relived as clients go through termination of physical treatment. As pointed out before, doctor-patient relationships are very prone to become saturated with transferential feelings, thoughts and fantasies. These ideas can hark back to earlier developmental epochs and the patient may use the transference as a vehicle for reliving these earlier periods of life in a more satisfying manner. If the body-worker is aware of this potentiality, much good can be done. The following case illustrates how a termination brought on by a job relocation, placed a strain on the patient's *object constancy*. Fortunately the doctor handled the situation empathically and professionally and all was well.

Case example: Beth and Termination

Beth was a 54-year-old woman who had been seeing Joyce, a naprapath, for a year for work on nagging pain in the sacral area. The pain had abated considerably, but Beth still came for "tune up" treatments every two weeks.

Beth had just gone through a painful divorce and, although she was highly invested in her children and grandchildren, she had few other outlets for her energies. She had not pursued a career. Consequently, it seemed that she had become very connected to Joyce, often confiding in her in the course of a treatment, sharing with her the joys and sadness of her life. It was as if Joyce, a naprapath, was being used in some ways, as a psychological counselor. Joyce did not feel put upon by this and did her best to listen and give support.

Eventually, however, a wonderful opportunity opened up for Joyce, a chance at professional development she could not pass up. It would mean she would have to leave the clinic where she was seeing Beth. Fortunately, Joyce was aware that Beth was relying on her in important ways, that there was a relationship that went well beyond a simple treatment. It was a relationship that could not be easily replaced with a standard referral. One could even argue that Joyce had become a selfobject for Beth and that if she should terminate the relationship too abruptly that Beth might deteriorate, both psychologically and physically, as a result.

Therefore, Joyce was careful to provide extensive opportunities for Beth to talk about the change. Joyce provided a referral to someone who she knew was very good and empathic. She offered to see Beth on a once-a-month basis, monitoring Beth's situation, and was ready to intervene should there be signs of disorganization or distress. Joyce's response, although she is not a counselor, is one that is sensitive to the emotional aspects of the patient's life and to the relationship. It is never just treatment. There is always an emotional side to the relationship, and one ignores this aspect at the risk of detriment to the patient's well-being.

Now we can perhaps see how the ways in which the individual may have traversed this era of self discovery and self definition during the first three years of life have become encoded into the body—into habitual ways of moving, posturing and habitual modes of relating to one's body and the bodies of others. We can also perhaps see how these modes may become lifelong issues—issues that manifest themselves in the process of body-work.

CHAPTER 7

Heinz Kohut: Narcissism and the Body

The human being is continually developing along multiple developmental lines. We saw in the previous section how one of those developmental lines is that of separation-individuation, having to do with an emerging sense of one's separateness and connectedness to others. We also saw how impasses, fixations and derailings of this process are embodied. We heard, for example, that for Mahler, "the trunk is the midwife to differentiation," meaning that as the infant gains control over her trunk muscles she becomes more able to separate herself physically and thus psychologically from her mother. Later, as a body-worker works on the trunk of the patient's body, it might be that thoughts, fantasies and feelings having to do with differentiation might surface.

In this section we take a similar approach with the developmental line of narcissism, the evolution of self esteem and all that is associated with it. There is a large literature on self esteem, but we will focus here on the ideas of Heinz Kohut whose theory explicitly links narcissistic vicissitudes to psychosomatic issues. First, we will examine Kohut's theory; then we will examine how these issues may manifest in body-work.

Kohut's Theory

Diagram 4 gives a very simplified outline of Kohut's theory. It is a radical compression of his very complex ideas expressed in several books (Kohut, 1971, 1977). It is important to remember that Kohut's is a psychodynamic theory and therefore much of this developmental process and its sequelae are unconscious.

Diagram 4: Kohut's Theory

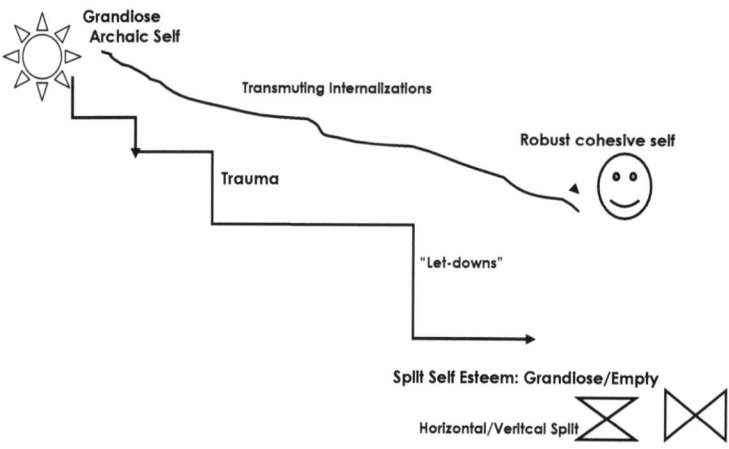

According to Kohut, we start life with a *"grandiose archaic self,"* a sense of ourselves that is omnipotent and wonderfully powerful. This sense of grandiosity is sustained by the tender, attentive care of our parents who provide, in addition to our physical needs, the three *selfobject* needs of *mirroring, idealization* and *merger and twinning.* The word *"selfobject"* is used by Kohut to suggest that self and other are psychologically fused, rather similar to the symbiotic stage of Mahler. As long as these three selfobject needs are in good supply, then the sense of self is sustained and energized. One feels enlivened and "together." As to the selfobject needs, they have the following meanings.

Mirroring refers to being accurately and empathically reflected in the other's eyes, language and behavior. When we are well mirrored we feel well held, deeply understood and this helps hold us together.

Idealization and merger refers to the feelings of intensely admiring another and at the same time believing oneself to be combined with that admired other and therefore partaking of their wonderful, seemingly magical powers.

Finally, **twinning** involves the feelings and thoughts associated with the idea that one has found another person who is one's twin, who is just like you in vitally important ways. One has a matching partner, a "running mate," and this helps consolidate and strengthen one's self esteem.

If these three selfobject needs are in reasonably abundant supply, then the self esteem is sustained. Inevitably, however, life's ups and downs result in interruptions of the supply, in letdowns. Others may not reflect us accurately, or they may turn out to be imperfect, to have feet of clay. Also, we may discover that our "twin" is different from us in important ways.

If these interruptions in the supply of selfobject needs are not too great and are not traumatic, then we are able to adjust. Through a process of what Kohut calls "transmuting internalizations" we learn how to soothe ourselves and maintain a robust self esteem. If we are "let down" gradually, in small increments, we are able to hold ourselves together and we retain our ideals and ambitions. We are also unlikely to develop psychosomatic illnesses (imaginary, symbolic illnesses) that symbolize our fear of falling to pieces, of losing our self esteem.

If, on the other hand, these selfobject needs are traumatically interrupted, then the result is a subjective sense that we are falling to pieces. This results in all sorts of panic reactions as the person attempts to hold themselves together—perhaps by becoming angry, by regressing to an earlier stage of development, turning to drugs, obsessive sexual activity, withdrawal, grandiosity or depression. Many times the narcissistic fragmentation (the sense of falling to pieces) shows up in bodily disturbances. Many physical ailments can be psychosomatic, resulting from the patient's feelings of fragmentation.

The following case shows how a body-worker making a simple, well-timed comment deepened the power of her treatment. Among other things, it shows how the simple process of mirroring can facilitate treatment.

Case Vignette: "Papa, why are you smoking?"   *Bill, a 55-year-old man, six foot two and weighing in at 250 pounds was trying to quit smoking. He was coming to the doctor for auricular therapy to help in this. In his conversations with the doctor, Bill shared that he was interested in starting Kung Fu classes and psychotherapy. He mentioned that his* *motivation to quit smoking had been deepened when his grandson had said to him, "Papa, why are you smoking?"*

A week or so later as the doctor was doing auricular therapy, she said quietly into Bill's ear, "Papa, why are you smoking?"

At this, he teared up as deep feelings surged to awareness. Later as Bill got ready to leave he said, "Thanks, Doc, for saying what you said. You remember everything I say!"

This vignette also demonstrates the potency of the relationship and listening. By remembering something significant that was said by Bill, the body-worker helped cement the bond of relationship and increased Bill's motivation. Such remembering also may help the strengthening of the patient's self-structure.

These processes can have terrific importance for body-workers in two ways.

First, some physical problems the body-worker encounters may trace back to narcissistic vulnerabilities in the patient. From conversation with the patient, the body-worker may be able to develop some ideas as to how narcissistic setbacks in the patient's life can lead to a worsening of the symptoms. Together with the patient, the body-worker may, if it feels appropriate and timely, develop with the patient some ideas about coping with setbacks to one's self esteem.

Secondly, the body-worker may find that the patient with narcissistic vulnerabilities responds strongly with a narcissistic transference onto them. This means that the patient may turn unconsciously to the body-worker for selfobject needs—mirroring, idealization and merger and twinning. They will expect the body-worker to actively empathize with them, to be admirable and to be just like them in important ways. When these selfobject needs are not met, a person with narcissistic vulnerabilities will disintegrate and manifest the symptoms mentioned above; sometimes they will somatize and symptoms will worsen or return. It is important to recall that many of these needs are met through non-verbal modes. Empathy, deep understanding, is often communicated through touch. Thus, patients with narcissistic issues may come for treatment of bodily issues with an unstated expectation to be understood without words, through touch. For many patients, the body-work session may be one island in their life where they experience narcissistic integrity. If this is the case, these vicissitudes in the treatment process may have more dramatic impacts on the patient with narcissistic issues than on patients who do not have narcissistic issues—patients who have a robust and cohesive sense of self.

For example, a patient who has narcissistic vulnerabilities may react to a change in the appointment schedule in some of the ways mentioned above. Her symptoms may worsen. She may become very angry or act out in some way, either in her personal life or in their relationship to the body-worker. She may get in a fight, get drunk, withdraw, become depressed, all in a frenzied attempt to shore up some cohesive sense of self. In relation to the body-worker, she may act out in various ways. She may miss sessions, show up late, forget checks, act upon the worker in such ways as to elicit low self esteem. Once the body-worker understands these reactions not as random or undetermined, but as panicked responses of an individual who is very afraid of losing her sense of self and is attempting to hold herself together, perhaps even trying, through her actions, to let the body-worker know how she feels.

This following case demonstrates that narcissistic issues can come in multiple forms. Sometimes narcissism can come with a charming seductive front, while at others it presents a brittle cool exterior and a sense of entitlement accompanied by a sensitivity to rejection and slights.

Case: Demands for Special Treatment: *Iris, 65, came to the office with a wide array of complaints- pain and joint stiffness in the hip, shoulder and neck and disturbed sleep. Emotionally, she was quite depressed. Interpersonally, she was lonely and often difficult. The body-worker found her confusing. At one moment, Iris was very grateful for any relief, and the next she was accusing the therapist of harming her in some way, even though the procedure had been light and low stress.*

Iris was also prone to behave in a very entitled manner, often demanding special treatment, asking for sessions at unusual times or at very short notice and becoming very irritated when her special requests were not granted. At the same time, Iris was often quite generous, sometimes bringing gifts of food, chocolates and gourmet breads for the body-worker to enjoy. The body-worker felt buffeted one way and then the next by Iris's paradoxical behaviors. She also felt anxious; for Iris shared that she was quite ready, willing and able to sue people by whom she felt wronged.

The body-worker tried to keep a steady hand, both physically and emotionally, during the treatment. She was available but professional, and in her behavior was able to provide reassurance to Iris that she was not aiming to exploit her. Also, while keeping her time and professional boundaries clear, she did not retaliate to Iris's entitled demeanor and requests for special treatment.

Eventually, after six months, it was as if the storm passed, as if the body-worker had passed several tests that Iris had been setting for her. As this happened, Iris started to have more focal responses to the body-work. She shared that she felt her whole life had been like a prison and that she had no friends. She felt the body-worker had opened a window for her and she could finally see light and the possibility of escape. She felt grateful for the help that the body-worker had given her.

Soon after, she shared two dreams she had. In one, she was locked in a prison and screaming. In the other, her mother was choking her. As she shared these dreams she remembered being beaten by her siblings and being physically punished by her mother in terrifying ways. "It's really coming to the surface now!" she declared at the end of one of these sessions. The body-worker coined the term "Bad Mother Syndrome" to describe the situation where a patient has seemingly internalized a toxic, hateful and abusive relationship with the mother in her body. The body-worker also concluded that in order to achieve relief of Iris's physical problems she would have to also empathically and sympathetically resonate with her memories, thoughts and feelings as they surfaced during the body-work.

CHAPTER 8

Somatization: A Fairbairnian Model

The term "somatization" refers to the process whereby thoughts, ideas, feelings, fantasies, impulses and wishes, in fact any mental process, manifest themselves in the body.

Somatization is different from the stress disorders because stress disorders result from alterations in the autonomic nervous system that are perhaps somewhat better understood. We are fairly familiar with the notion that stress can alter our nervous and hormonal system, increasing our blood pressure, altering our digestion and affecting our muscle tone, and that these changes can result in disease.

Somatization disorders overlap with stress-related disorders and the boundaries between the two are currently indeterminate since much is being learned about neuropeptides--chemical messengers secreted in the brain and picked up by receptor sites throughout the body, affecting the functioning of all our bodily organs. (Pert,1999)

More "psychological" in nature are the somatizations that are similar to the ones induced under hypnosis by Charcot and studied by Janet (1889/1973) and Breuer and Freud (1885/2000). Gathered together under this category would be some of the "hysterical" conditions of nineteenth century psychiatry. Often, these disorders are metaphoric in nature. A person who feels guilty about masturbation might develop an hysterical paralysis of his hand,

A person who saw things she wishes she had not seen might develop hysterical blindness. A person who could not stand to be in the presence of someone toward whom she harbored intense, painful and perhaps conflicted feelings, might develop hysterical fainting fits. These conditions are different from specifically stress-related disorders such as high blood pressure or from the ways in which blood sugar level is affected by social processes (see Pelletier,2003; Benson, 2000; Minuchin 1978). Of course these conditions will overlap. These situations that give rise to stress-related conditions will also affect secretions of neuropeptides and will at the same time create ideas that can manifest in physical conditions. The clinician has a monumental task in unraveling the complex causal matrices in such cases.

There are many theories in the psychodynamic paradigm, but that of WRD Fairbairn (1952) will serve us very well here to elucidate several of the dynamics involved in some forms of somatization.

Figure 5 gives a schematic diagram of developments in the mind- he calls it his "endopsychic model."

Figure 5: Fairbairn's Endopsychic Model

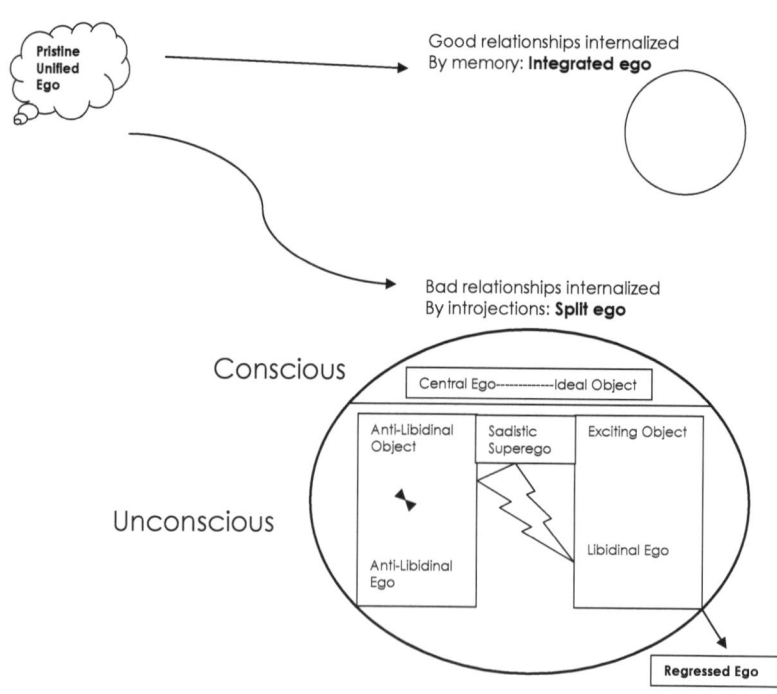

We start off life with a 'pristine unified ego' which is an ego structure that is, as yet "unmarked" with any memories or experience. Our basic drive or motivation is to seek other people and have satisfying relationships with them. If these relationships are, on the whole, satisfactory then we follow the pathway along the top of the model and simply internalize these relational experiences (that is take them into our mind) in the form of memories. Memories form relatively flexible, relatively adaptable and integrated units in the mind. Thus the more the personality is built from memories resulting from satisfying interactions with others the more likely the mind is to stay together, to adapt and the less likely is the person to go to pieces or fall apart, other things being equal. Memories are retrievable, modifiable and integrable.

On the other hand, if the infant, toddler or child is unfortunate enough to have unpleasant relationships, these are not internalized (taken into the mind) in the form of memories but as *introjections*, meaning the offending experience is taken in as a whole, metaphorically, as if the experience is swallowed whole. When the experience is internalized in this drastic emergency form (perhaps so that, in fantasy, it can be controlled), the experience is not integrated so fully with the rest of the personality. These introjects act rather like semi-autonomous sub-personalities in the unconscious mind. We, thus, end up with the internal arrangement depicted in the lower right hand of the figure.

We can see that the personality, instead of being a relatively integrated matrix of memories, is a dissociated group of sub-personalities of "objects" and "egos" (selves and others) that are introjects of troubling images of others and aspects of one's self that were in relation to those others.

At the heart of the personality is the libidinal ego, which is the remnant of the original pristine unified ego that still yearns for close contact with others and the world. This ego, however, is linked to an introject called the exciting object, which does not satisfy, but only torments, offering, but never fulfilling, promises of relational satisfaction. This is an introjection of past experiences with others that had this tantalizing, teasing quality.

The libidinal ego is also under attack from the two introjects that result from the hostile aspects of relationships to others--the anti-libidinal ego and the anti-libidinal object. Both of these gang up on the libidinal ego as the "internal saboteur." They aim at sabotaging any attempts it might make at relating to others. This sabotage is done by the internal saboteur as if to protect the libidinal ego from further insult and injury as if to say, "We are protecting you for your own good," or, "Do not hope for too much. Do not love. It will only end up badly."

The exciting object will often result in the individual being haunted by intense longings and frustrations they cannot quite articulate, and often one will act out this internal scenario in relationships with others that have this tantalizing, tormenting quality. In addition, the internal saboteur will sabotage, undermine and destroy the individual's attempts to establish positive relationships with others and their world.

Thus an individual with a pronounced internal saboteur may have a strong "negative therapeutic reaction." Meaning that, as his life starts to improve as a result of an intervention, say, therapy, massage, or a naprapathic treatment, he unconsciously sets about undermining it in some way. He may seek out an injurious experience or relationship, or perhaps internally, that is, within his own mind, through the attacks on the libidinal ego carried out by the internal saboteur. In extreme cases, where the internal saboteur is especially virulent and violent, its actions can result in profound emotional paralysis, disorganization or numbness.

Clearly, all this internal activity can take up a lot of energy and not much is left over for dealings with the outside world. Thus, we see the conscious part of the mind, comprised of what Fairbairn calls the *"Ideal Object"* and the *"Central Ego."* These are what is left over of the mind once the splitting up into internal objects has taken place. The central ego and ideal object form together a mask, a sort of false self with which the individual confronts the world. This mask is, as we can see, disconnected from the libidinal ego, the personality's source of energy, thus the individual in this schizoidal or split state easily fatigues and often feels out of touch with herself or has difficulty feeling real or making authentic spontaneous contact with others.

This internal arrangement can also have multiple physical effects that the body-worker should be aware of. For example, we have worked with several patients who presented with various forms of chronic pain syndrome that had eluded a stable diagnosis by several physicians and these, we believe, exemplified this internal scenario.

Sandra, a client in psychological counseling helps illustrate these dynamics and, in addition, shows how Fairbairn's scheme can be used to explain an array of psychosomatic complaints.

Case Vignette: Chronic Pain as a Result of Bad Introjects

Sandra, a petite 54-year-old woman, arrived at the office with a battery-powered device she activated every few minutes to alleviate her chronic pain, which she experienced throughout her body, but most seriously and disablingly in her legs. She was very lonely and isolated, and she had a job where she would often be traumatized by angry outbursts from her boss. She had few friends, few hobbies and lived in a neighborhood that frightened her. She was quite challenging to work with since she took quite a while to "warm up" and to start talking. She often felt as though the counselor was simply out to "suck her dry of money."

Counseling proceeded haltingly, for it was quite difficult for Sandra to get in touch with her feelings and to "warm up" and engage in the process. She also found it painful to talk about her childhood memories, often blanking out in what seemed to be spontaneous hypnotic trances. Despite these and other difficulties, we were able to examine Sandra's life and establish a working alliance, albeit a rather fragile and brittle one.

Perhaps the most interesting feature was that over the first year or so of counseling Sandra's pain diminished so dramatically that she no longer needed the electrical stimulation device and had taken up the hobby of walking. She had found a friend and together they would go on long strolls though the forest preserves. An analysis of what had happened from a Fairbairnian perspective would be as follows: Sandra had a very bad relationship with her mother, extending back, in her memory and estimation, to the earliest stages of her life. She believed her mother hated her; not with the hot hatred one feels in the midst of a passionate fight but with an enduring cold hatred, sustained over decades. Sandra had internalized this hatred as an introjection. She, thus, had a hating mother inside her mind, an internalized object continually attacking her libidinal ego, interrupting her well-being and stopping her from establishing satisfying relationships with others. The counselor hypothesized that Sandra's introjected hating mother was so virulent and highly energized that it also affected her body- causing her chronic pain. As the satisfactory relationship with the therapist was established, and as the violence of the introjected mother was moderated through remembering and working through, so its negative impacts were reduced and resulted in her libidinal ego finding attachments with others in reality. It also resulted in a reduction of bodily complaints, especially the chronic pain.

The case of Sandra illustrates the possible utility of the Fairbairn object relations model in explaining and, even treating, chronic pain when physical causes are difficult to discern. Posited here is the possibility that such pain could result from intrapsychic dynamics rooted in the introjection of traumatic relationships.

This following case illustrates how the release of locked energy in the body can release an appetite for life (in the Fairbairnian system this appetite would be called the libidinal ego) and how this can cause the patient to come to sessions with new problems, albeit more positive problems—problems that come from having raised one's life expectations. In other words, they are good problems.

Case: Career Counseling

Joanna came to see a naprapath complaining of severe pain down her arms. She was 50 years old and had just taken an offer of early retirement from her position as a baggage handler with an airline. The decision to take the offer of early retirement was prompted, in part, by her arm pain.

After four visits to the naprapath, the pain had almost gone—90% relief. The work the naprapath had done had been quite straightforward, involving "stripping" the median nerve of the arm of adhesions so it was freer to carry out is functions. On the fifth visit Joanna said, "I wish I hadn't retired!"

"Yes, what are you going to do with the next half of your life?" asked the naprapath.

"I have no idea! My husband says I'm driving him crazy around the house all the time."

"Try this," said the naprapath. "Think of work you would like to do so much you would do it even if you didn't get paid."

Joanna thought for a while and after musing about how she liked to help people but not sick or depressed people, came up with the job of concierge. Her eyes lit up and then she immediately gave up, citing the depressed economy.

"Don't worry so much about that. Follow your passion, look into classes, courses. Check it out at least," encouraged the naprapath.

"Yeah, no harm in doing that," assented Joan, and the life came back in her face.

This case vignette illustrates several concepts that are crucial to body-workers—that the increase in bodily functioning leads to increases in functionality on many fronts and these often present problems of adjustment for the patient. It is important that the body-worker be sensitive to these adaptations and proffer his support in the direction of growth and expansion of function.

Note also how Joanna's "internal saboteur" emerged quickly in response to her opening up and excitement (her "libidinal ego"). Note how quite simply, the naprapath's response of encouragement was enough, at least in this case, to overcome this attempt at self negation. We will see in several of the cases in the upcoming section on social systems and the body how this selfsame process of sabotage can operate between persons.

In some instances the client may be dominated and terrorized by an internalized bad object. This can lead to the experiencing of anxiety attacks. It is as if the internalized object is a bully that attacks and frightens the libidinal ego every time it makes an attempt at embracing life in an expansive affirming way. The following case vignette gives an idea of how Antonio, a personal trainer, joined forces with the libidinal ego to help it find a way out into the world.

Case: "Allies"

Gladys came to Antonio stating that she wanted to build her confidence in herself and do some strength training. In conversations between sets, she revealed that she grew up in an abusive family environment and that she had taken up the role of protector of the other, younger kids, often having to steel herself against the fear that she felt on a chronic basis. Just recently, however, she had been visiting a psychiatrist for "panic attacks", attacks of trembling and fear that she could not comprehend. If we recall chapter one of this book, we can recall that is not uncommon with traumatized individuals. They can bear up under the strain for so long and then their defenses may give way, exhausted, and the underlying feelings flood forth. Antonio seemed to intuitively understand that this was what was happening and offered that he was going to challenge her with exercises and that these would push her close to exhaustion. He, however would support her and push her through until she got stronger. It was as though an alliance was being cast between Antonio and the beleaguered childhood self of Gladys. She seemed to take it that way. Together they would fight the enemy, the symbolic enemy of the stress and strain of the exercise, and she would get stronger and gain in confidence and courage. The work with the weights and the exercise became a sort of psychodrama for her in which she could push through the abuse of her childhood into confident contact with the adult world.

The following case demonstrates how several of these theories can conflate to provide powerful explanations for the seemingly everyday phenomenon of giving up smoking and working on a "bad back."

Case: Bill and the Anxious Liberation of Libido

Bill, a 62-year-old male, six foot three and weighing 263 pounds, came to treatment to give up smoking, using auricular therapy. He was highly motivated to change and took up walking and cycling. He ceased smoking and started to feel much better.

At this point a new problem emerged. Bill complained that while his sexual desire had increased, he was having painful pelvic muscle spasms during sex. The body-worker worked on relaxing Bill's very tense psoas muscle and Bill had a complex reaction to this. On the one hand he cried out "Exactly!" when the naprapath worked on the psoas, letting her know that this was the core of his problem. On the other hand, he felt a deep sense of despair about his life—a despair that he felt he had been nursing for a long time, a sense of a life unlived, of potentialities not realized.

If we are familiar with the theories of Reich, Lowen and Fairbairn, the case of Bill is not at all surprising. It can be interpreted as follows. The cessation of smoking, combined with the supportive work of the naprapath and exercise, leads to an increase in Bill's libido (to use the old-fashioned but felicitous term for 'lust for life'). This in turn leads to an increase in sexual desire. Immediately, however, this increase encounters what Reich would call "character armor"—tight muscles that prevent energetic flow in the body. This character armor, linked with what Lowen calls "pleasure anxiety" can be regarded as a rigid encasement of despair. As it gives way, both pleasure and remembered despair will break into consciousness.

Psychodynamically, smoking is often understood as an identification with a depressed mother. As the individual gives up smoking, it can be seen as a relinquishing of his identification with the depression he encountered in his mother. This disidentification can be extremely difficult. Often it will activate negative spoiling introjects parallel to Fairbairn's "internal saboteur" that aims to destroy the libidinal ego's attempts to connect lovingly and meaningfully with the world. In the case of Bill, these introjects were embodied via his psoas and its related spasms.

We thus can understand Bill's forward progress as an attempt to live his life outside the influence of depressing and sabotaging introjects. Fortunately, the naprapath was able to be a supportive companion in this enterprise. Bill also shows us that emotional growth can indeed be a lifelong process.

We hope we have demonstrated some of the rich possibilities that exist in the connections between theories of psychological development and bodily processes. Of course, the list of developmental theories is very long and we will not examine all that they have to offer here. However, one more theory is worthy of a special mention and readers are encouraged to explore it further. Daniel Stern, in his epochal work *The Interpersonal World of the Infant* (2000), presents a model of the self which we believe fits very nicely with the theory of Kohut, while calling into question some of Mahler's concepts.

Stern's theory is rich and complex, and we will only offer a simplified version here. He argues that there are four aspects to self-experience: cohesion (the sense of being together and integrated), affectivity (the feelings, emotions and passions we have and their intensity), continuity (the sense we have of "going on being", of existing through time) and agency (the sense that we can make things happen in our world). In addition, he posits that there are four levels or types of self-experience at which these four aspects operate: emergent (the aspects of self that are just coming into being), core (the aspects of self that we accept of being invariant parts of our identities), interpersonal (the aspects of ourselves that are related to others) and verbal (which includes the ways in which we construct symbolic narratives of our selves). Each of these will develop continuously as we grow and each will intertwine with bodily processes. We highly recommend this work to all therapists. It is still having impacts on the worlds of psychotherapy and related fields decades after its publication.

Section III
Social Systems and the Body

So often, especially in a culture that places a high premium on individuality, we see illness and disease as lying inside the individual. However an alternative perspective, one that is based on a family systems perspective, informs us that illness and disease could emanate from group dynamics, especially if that powerful group is one's family.

CHAPTER 9

Bodily Reactions to Group Phenomena and the Body in the Family

The following case demonstrates the common sense notion that we can carry emotional issues, stemming from our family and other groups we inhabit, in our bodies. The body-worker will often have to take these factors into account if treatment gains are to be made and maintained.

Case: Karen, overloaded:

Karen, 53 years old, came to the naprapath complaining of "pain from head to toe!" Tests revealed a stenosis in the lumbar region. She spoke very quietly, speaking of how she had to manage the entire household, always caring for others, especially her aging and ill mother.

The body-worker worked on Karen's trapezius muscles and neck. As she did so Karen shared, "This body just needs to scream!" It was as if she was filled with decades of pent up rage, as if she wanted to "blow her top." Interestingly, as if in a metaphor, she had a mild stroke the previous year. The body-worker listened to Karen's emotional outpourings and Karen started to show improvement. She complained that her previous doctor was "not so good," there was too little contact.

Sometimes as she stood up she would state, "I just want to scream!" The body-worker, in conversation, explored with Karen ways to let it all out productively, and perhaps do more things just for herself. Karen was open to these ideas but found it very hard to follow through. She felt she had so many responsibilities at home.

Diagram 6 is a diagram of a group from a psychodynamic perspective.

Diagram 6: Schematic Diagram of a Group from a Group-as-a-Whole Perspective

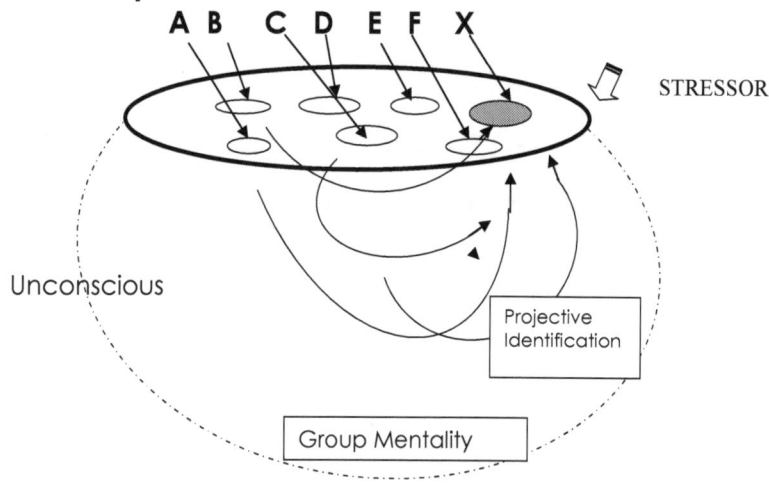

We can see that the group has seven members A, B, C, D, E, F, and X. The ellipse encircling the members designates the boundaries of the group. Above each member we can imagine the individual's conscious mind and under each individual we can imagine the individual's unconscious mind. The broken line hanging under the ellipse designates the group boundary and encloses the group mentality--the unconscious "mind" of the group. (I explore the dynamics and application of this model of groups in my book *Imaginary Groups* [2005].)

How does this conception of the group relate to the somatization? Briefly, when a stress impacts the group (and the stress can come from internal or external sources) we can expect an array of emotions will be stimulated in its members. Many of these feelings will be painful and difficult to manage. They will, therefore, be dealt with through a battery of defense mechanisms—repression, denial, dissociation, splitting and so on into members' individual unconscious minds. When, however, we are in a group, we have an additional line of defense. We can send, using the defense mechanism of projective identification, unwanted parts of ourselves into the unconscious of the group--the group mentality. Thus, if a stress should hit or press upon a group, the situation depicted in diagram 6 obtains.

Members of the group, to varying degrees, experience uncomfortable emotions, fear, grief or excitement. They then dissociate from these emotions and the accompanying thoughts and feelings and projectively identify them into the group mentality. Once there, these unwanted emotions can, in imagination, travel to several other locations.

First, they might be located in another group which is then viewed as containing these unwanted elements. Many intergroup and organizational dynamics can be explained as stemming from these dynamics.

Second, these unwanted pieces may occupy an imaginary space in the group, operating like a "presence," sometimes in, sometimes above, sometimes around the group. Groups using this form of defense mechanism may feel the presence and influence of "entities" or "forces" that are difficult to identify or describe. These "presences" are very powerful, sometimes crushing the group spirit like an imaginary secret police or encircling their sphere of action like a surrounding force-field.

Third, the group may unconsciously elect one of its members to become a container for these unwanted feelings—a repository, a form of scapegoat. Who is selected as a repository depends on several factors. If one is a singleton in the group -- the only woman, the oldest, the youngest, the only African American, etc. -- one is more liable to become a repository for the group's unwanted feelings. The feelings and projected parts of the self are distributed along the lines of very simple-minded prejudices. For example, the only woman in a group will perhaps be unconsciously pressured to carry "feminine" parts as defined by conventional stereotypes, the youngest member may become a repository of feelings, thoughts and impulses stereotypically expected of the young. Repositories thus "elected" (for this selection process, while powerful, is mostly unconscious) are treated very ambivalently by the group. On the one hand, they are often disliked by the group. At the same time, because they are serving an important function for the group, by containing its unwanted parts, they are needed and, paradoxically valued, by the group.

Persons of low status are liable to become repositories for

unwanted thoughts and feelings in the group. It is as if low status individuals or sub-groups do not have enough counter-power to thwart the projective identifications of those of higher status. Thus, for example, a low ranking assistant or secretary will often be used to hold anxieties and concerns that in reality belong to the whole office or organization.

People who occupy positions at or near the boundaries of an organization are vulnerable to becoming a repository. Thus a receptionist, a compliance officer, an intern, a new recruit or those who are soon to retire are likely to be used as containers for the undesirable. The person at the boundary is metaphorically on the skin of the group and carries all the intense meaning that the skin carries for any organism. At the boundary, the person is privy to tensions operating inside and outside the group. Often one's loyalties can be divided between those inside and outside. These are among the factors that set up the boundary person as a target for projective identifications.

An individual's personality will affect their likelihood of becoming a repository and the types of projections they are liable to introject and live out for the group. Some people are well-prepared, as it were, to be rebels. Perhaps they have a family background and a personal history which has given them a taste for and a training in rebellion. Thus, should the group go though some experiences that stimulate a rebelliousness that most members are uncomfortable with, the aforementioned member with a "schooling" in rebellion will perhaps emerge as a container of the group's rebellious feelings. Historical examples of this can be found in Erikson's analyses of Martin Luther, Hitler and Ghandi (1963,1968,1993). There was widespread antipathy toward the corruption of the papacy in the early 16th century. Martin Luther had a history of anger at his father. Erikson argues that Luther's personal history set him up perfectly for the religious rebellion that was at the start of Protestantism.

One can be set up for a repository function in a group by virtue of one's designated role in the group. The term "mother" carries with it many expectations regarding how one is supposed to behave, as do the roles of "police officer," "accountant," "counselor," "receptionist." These labels have enormous power in allocating certain types of thoughts, feelings and fantasies to certain individuals or groups. Oftentimes the power of these role designations is overlooked. Zimbardo's famous "prison experiment" (2004) serves as a reminder of just how powerful these forces can be.

We thus can have a situation operating in a group, an office, or an organization, where there are extremely powerful feelings operating in the unconscious of the group and that are being located, projectively identified, absorbed by certain vulnerable individuals, sub-groups or even groups. These powerful emotions, group emotions, affect not only the mind of those who are containing them but also their bodies. Thus in addition to the stress-related illnesses and disturbances of life in a stressed group, we may see, in certain individuals who have become repositories, somatization disorders that often capture metaphorically the pressures the group is finding problematic.

Perhaps the following examples will help illustrate some of these dynamics.

Case Vignette: Derek, *"I've had it up to here!"*:

Derek was a 45-year-old African American man who was dean of students at an inner city college. His job was very stressful, especially since there was a widespread attitude in the college that he was the "go to" guy when it came to dealing with discipline problems. In addition he was being given very little support, either moral or in terms of personnel, from upper management. His staff and budget had been reduced and his capacity to cope with the situations he faced as a professional was being seriously challenged. Derek was a quiet man, not prone to complain or openly express his anger; he was much more likely to "gut it out." And that, interestingly, is what happened. After a year or so of this near impossible work situation, he developed a condition that was diagnosed as inflammatory bowel disease. He was suffering and looked very poorly when we spoke to him. After he described his situation we ventured that the metaphor "full of shit" captured both his physical condition and his primary process feelings about the college where he was working. After some careful consideration and coming to the realization that his work situation was very unlikely to change, he decided to quit his job and work for an organization that was not so psychotoxic.

While we cannot rule out many other possible contributors to Derek's condition--genetics, diet, trauma--we are left with the deep conviction that his physical condition was stimulated, not only by these and the stress of his position, but also by a group-forced psychogenic process wherein the organization unconsciously asked him to contain and carry much of its "inflammatory shit"—processes it was unable or unwilling to examine verbally; processes that then are more likely to be somatized by a vulnerable repository. Derek was set up to become a repository of the organization's unconscious issues by virtue of his role, his personality and his singleton status.

The following case illustrates the complexity of the personality when we take on these multiple perspectives, for it illustrates how personality, the body, life stage development, organizational and familial issues can all intertwine in a "Gordian Knot" that manifests as a physical problem resulting from an accident at work.

Case Vignette: Brian, not enough backup:

Brian was a 36-year-old man who had problems in finding his niche in life. For the last five years he had been working as a general office assistant—a position considerably below his competence level. He had graduate credits in political science, but he had problems finding an "anchor" and completing his studies. Additionally, he was not treated with respect at his job. He felt beaten down by his bosses and was filled with feelings of impotent rage. Bioenergetically, it made sense that his pelvis was locked, held tight by a taut psoas muscle. This would jam up his pelvis and prevent the free expression of his sexual energy, both erotic and aggressive. He mentioned, in fact, that he was so depressed by his work situation that he had not had sex with his wife for over a year. One day he was filing some boxes in the office and ruptured a lumbar disc and strained two others.

Again with Brian, as Derek, we cannot rule out a host of causative factors. One that remains is that his work situation, where he was serving as a scapegoat and filling up with dissociated helpless rage, was creating somatic tensions that made him vulnerable to a ruptured disc. In addition, Brian's family background as the youngest brother, preyed upon as a scapegoat by an alcoholic father and two disturbed older brothers, gave him a history and a preparation for playing this role. He now found himself in serious need of the "backing" or "rearing" that was lacking in both his family and his current work situation.

The following case is drawn from the literature on group dynamics and illustrates beautifully how everyday stresses and strains in work groups can manifest in the bodies of one or more the members.

Leroy Wells (1985) in an excellent article gives this example.

Case Vignette: Mr. W, Used as a repository:
Mr. W is a member of a research and development team that is under considerable pressure to come up with a technological innovation to help save the company. Mr. W is the oldest member of the team and has been cleverly and unconsciously maneuvered into the role of being the scapegoat, the reason the project would fail. Team members complained about Mr. W behind his back, and built the myth of his difficulty and incompetence. However, they would never confront him directly. In turn, Mr. W was unaware of the group's negative attitude toward him. He did, however, notice that he had been getting much more frequent migraine attacks.

Mr. W., being the oldest member, was in a way an ideal repository or target for the group's split-off fears of incompetence and shame. Ageism, operating here unconsciously, served to mark Mr. W, unawares, as the scapegoat. He also was somatizing, with migraine headaches. Interestingly, he was not consciously experiencing stress, although his group was under considerable pressure to perform. The migraines could have been induced by an activated sympathetic nervous system, but it is indeed interesting to hypothesize that some of the disabling migraines were group level somatizations that added, as it were, a physical vector to the scapegoating psychological dynamics.

Although very difficult to prove in an empirical fashion, this following case is a fascinating and provocative example of just how far the body might go in "metaphorizing" group dynamics.

Case Vignette: "Gall Bladder"
Senedra was an operating theater nurse who had recurrent problems with her gall bladder. She wondered aloud, half-discounting it as a crazy thought, if her work had anything to do with her chronic condition that puzzled many doctors.

In further conversations, it emerged that Senedra was a focal member of the nursing team. All the other members would come to her with their problems, both personal and professional. They would not talk to their supervisor because she would blame them for not "coming up with solutions." As a result, the team, growing increasingly bitter, would use Senedra as a repository for their frustrations.

Two tantalizing ideas surfaced. Could it be that Senedra's physical problems were related to these dynamics? Was she filling up with the bitterness or bile of the group? The gall bladder secretes bile salts which are used for digesting fat. Could it be that in "chewing the fat" with Senedra, her co-workers were overloading her gall bladder?

When asked, Senedra revealed that the role she was playing on the nursing team was not a new one for her. She had played this role in several other meaningful groups before, including her family.

This vignette shows how a physical symptom can sometimes be treated as a dream, sometimes as a social dream (Lawrence, 2007) and can yield useful hypotheses when subjected to even cursory levels of interpretation.

In addition, all of our acquaintances who work therapeutically with groups have noticed similar phenomena as feelings start to run high in groups—asthmatic attacks, dizziness, coughing fits, muscle cramps and so on that seem uncannily related to the group's here-and-now process.

The body-worker, thus, should be aware of the groups his patients inhabit and the extent to which their symptoms are related to these. He also would be well advised, if he wishes to take care of himself, to pay attention to the dynamics of the groups he inhabits.

Family Dynamics and the Body

Of course, the most influential group of which we are a member is the family group. As the following case illustrates, the family and its dynamics can be an extremely powerful force in the creation and maintenance of physical illness and will often play a powerful role in the treatment process. The body-worker who does not pay attention to such factors is perhaps compromising their effectiveness. Salvador Minuchin, in his fascinating book "Psychosomatic Families" (1978) gives a fascinating explanation of the multiple dynamisms and structures that underlie these processes. All illness which has a psychosomatic dimension also has a family systems component (Hazell, 2005).

The following cases illustrate how the same group dynamics we see operating in the institutional setting examined above operate at a high level of intensity and persuasiveness in families.

Case: Family Systems, Symptoms and Pain

Anne, a 38-year-old mother of two, came to Jackie, a naprapath, with a constellation of troubling problems: diabetes, chronic pain, fatigue, chest pains and obesity. Anne and Jackie formed a strong therapeutic alliance and Anne started to improve. The pain lifted, she became more energized and started to exercise and changed to a healthier nutritional regimen. She chose to use her new found energy and go on a much-needed vacation with a girlfriend.

At this point Anne's family, especially her mother and father, who would often accompany her to Jackie's office, started to complain that she was being foolish and selfish to go on vacation. They even started to develop symptoms as the vacation date approached. They used these symptoms as a way of engaging Anne, who seemed to have the role of family "nurse." Anne's mother suffered an attack of asthma on the day before her departure. Jackie intervened by telling the family that the vacation was an important aspect of Anne's treatment, that she needed to rest, relax and replenish. She even suggested that perhaps Anne was serving as a sort of container for family stress and that this might be contributing to Anne's debilitating conditions.

Interestingly, Anne herself was somewhat complicit in this arrangement; at times she seemed to balk at taking further steps into health as if the old family role sucked her back. At these times, Jackie would provide extra encouragement.

Jackie had the odd intuition that Anne was used as a sort of kidney or dialysis machine for the family. It was as if she took in all the toxicity from the family and had the unconsciously assigned task of purifying it. As she became healthier and healthier—losing weight, exercising and eating right—so the family had to reclaim the split-off parts they had projectively identified into Anne. As they did so, they also became physically more ill. The mother had to spend several days in hospital.

Jackie found that she, along with her MD partners, were working with the entire family system, moving the whole group toward improved health and psychosocial functioning. For example, when Anne wished to go out for a walk, or start an exercise regimen, her parents would quiz her, asking, "Why do you want to do that?" They would continually remind her of her her infirmities and her fragility, all this having the effect of undermining her confidence. One was reminded of the metaphor of crabs trying to escape from a bucket—as soon as one looked like it was about to get over the edge, the others would clasp it in their claws and pull it back into the confusional morass.

While some families are very distant from one another and have very little contact and offer one another minimal support, other families are very enmeshed and seem to have an unstated wish to stay together, no matter what this may cost in terms of the health of the individuals in the family. Often, this enmeshment can be understood as emanating from problems in separation individuation, as described in Mahler's theory.

The following vignette, shows how complicated mourning can become entrenched in an individual and in a family system. The body-work runs into resistances and sabotage as a result. The body-worker, confronts the family dynamic to good effect.

Case Vignette: Confrontation

Myrtle, 68 years old, was suffering from chronic, diffuse pain for which she was visiting the naprapath twice a week. She would complain that the music in the office sounded bad, "like dead people's music."

The naprapath, who felt in good contact with Myrtle, confronted her. "Perhaps you don't like the music because it helps you make contact with me—it is actually more of a life-giving, life-affirming music."

"Maybe," replied Myrtle, but her life persisted in its passive, inactive form. She rarely went out and had a very pessimistic, dark attitude regarding life and the future. She manifested most of the signs and symptoms of depression.

Her daughter, Laura, was also in treatment and was responding very well. However, Myrtle seemed to sabotage or question her daughter's health, asking her why she needed to exercise, go cycling, or take a dance class. Myrtle's depression was having a family systemic psychosomatic effect.

The naprapath recommended counseling for Myrtle, whom she felt was suffering from complicated mourning, perhaps for a long time. She also confronted Myrtle, asking her what she was going to do for the rest of her life, asking her if she felt any responsibility to Bert, her husband who was concerned about her pain, her depression and her inactivity. The body-worker felt that there were enough resources in the family and that her relationship with Myrtle was strong enough to take such a vigorous confrontation.

Slowly, step by step, Myrtle became more active and gradually accepted the increased activity level of her daughter, encouraged on the one hand by the naprapath and her husband; on the other, by the simple rewards and pleasures of living a more vibrant lifestyle in a more active family.

This vignette nicely illustrates the interaction of somatic problems, depression and family systems dynamics, and how the body-worker can intervene to judiciously question an enmeshment in the family that is involved in the persistence of these problems. The judgment as to whether and when to confront such dynamics and the manner in which to do it is a complex one. Such confrontations will usually stimulate anxiety and place a strain on the individual, the family and the relationship to the body-worker. Body-workers (and counselors) should consider these factors before offering such interventions. In addition, it is vitally important that the intervention is not a "hit and run" intervention, the body-worker or counselor should be available to assist in working through the adjustments that follow upon such confrontations or challenges.

The following vignette illustrates how a relatively transitional stress in a family issuing from a divorce might manifest in or be emotionally related to physical symptoms.

Case Vignette: Bracing

Brian, a 34-year old male, was coming to treatment for leg and back pain. When he laid on his back, he was so tense that he could not raise his leg.

The doctor, sensing that the tightness in his body was as if he was preparing for a shock, asked with a deliberate layering of meaning to her tone, "What are you bracing yourself for?"

Brian heard the double meaning and opened up. He talked about his divorce and how he was engaged in an unpleasant custody battle. He felt chronically sad and under stress, especially since his body pain prevented him from playing his favorite sport, soccer.

Following this ventilation of his feelings, his sense of foreboding and anxiety lifted somewhat and he became more able to raise his leg.

CHAPTER 10

Stress, Loss, Adaptation And The Body

Change is a constant and we have to adjust to changes psychologically and physiologically. In fact, these two categories are so intertwined that it is only for the convenience of exposition that we should separate them.

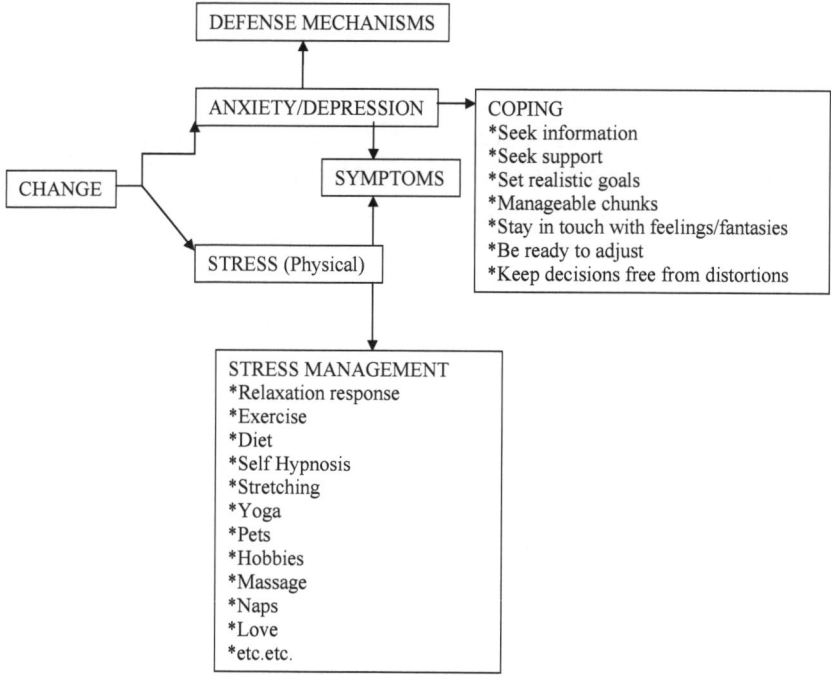

Diagram 7: A Model of Reactions to Change

Diagram 7 presents, in flow chart form, a simplified version of the human response to change. We can see that change brings on, to a greater or lesser extent, two categories of response: physiological, which we shall call "stress," and psychological. Psychological stress falls into two subtypes, anxiety (which is related to the loss of control we experience when things change) and depression (which is brought on by the loss that we experience when things change). The anxiety and depression can become painful and for that reason we mobilize our psychological defense mechanisms—unconscious psychological maneuvers aimed at reducing this pain, but at the cost of contact with reality. Or, we may respond to change by coping, by facing the reality of the situation, solving our problems and adjusting. We will return to these defenses and coping in chapter 12, "Personality Disorders in Everyday Practice."

Stress can be defined as the bodily reaction to change. A change in our environment (even a "positive" change, like a vacation) creates an array of physical responses called the FIGHT-FLIGHT-FREEZE response. Our body gears up very quickly to combat an enemy, to run away from danger or to stay stock still until the danger has passed. The fight-flight-freeze response is governed by the autonomic nervous system which operates in the "lower" brain centers automatically and, for the most part, beyond conscious control. This last factor is important. It means that it is possible for the fight-flight-freeze response to be activated without people necessarily being aware of it.

We see in the flow chart (Diagram 8) that when the organism perceives a change in its environment, the automatic nervous system activates the fight-flight-freeze response—a gamut of reflexive responses geared towards survival. Here is a list of some of the fight-flight- freeze responses.

FIGHT- FLIGHT- FREEZE RESPONSES
- increased pulse rate.
- increased blood pressure.
- pupil dilation.
- increased adrenalin secretion.
- slower digestion speeds.
- reduced skin temperature.
- increased sweating.

- dry mouth.
- increased muscle tension.

Diagram 8: The Stress Cycle

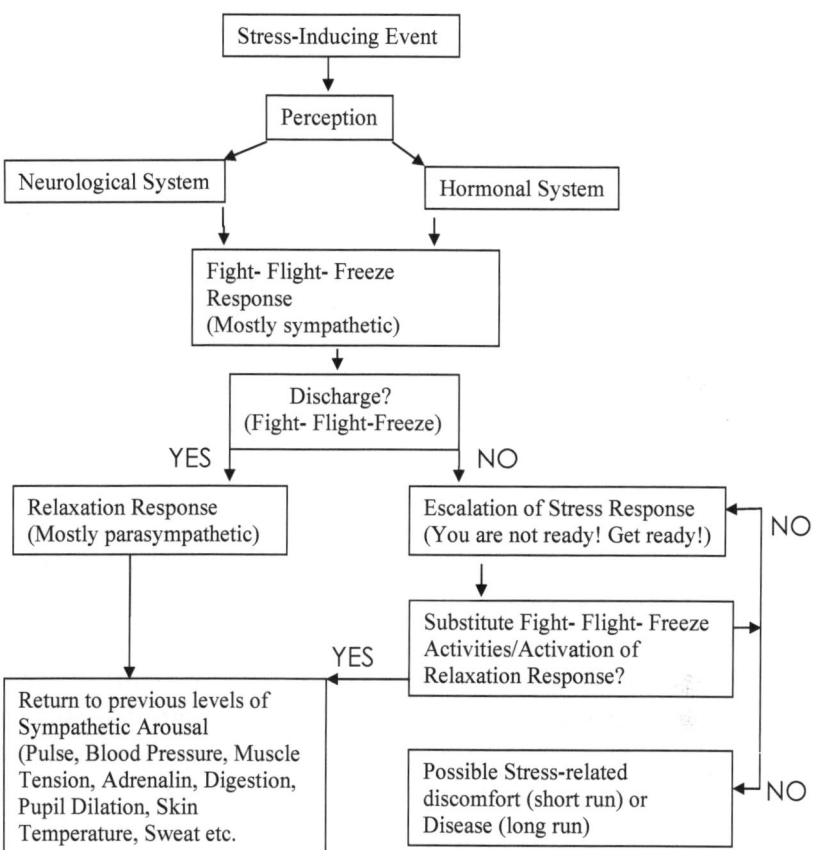

All of these are aimed to increase the likelihood that the individual will adapt to change and survive. If one is under attack, for example, why waste energy digesting food? You can do that later; better to send energy to the brain, heart, lungs and large muscles that are likely to be recruited in a survival effort.

Increased adrenalin will increase the power of muscles. Cool skin occurs because blood is withdrawn from the skin surface and sent to more central bodily locations, where it will do more good. Also, bleeding will be reduced if we are wounded. Sweating cools us down and makes us slippery prey. These arguments posit that the fight-flight- freeze responses are genetically programmed as a result of millions of years of evolution. Animals which did not have these were less likely to survive an attack and were "selected out" of the species.

Ancient though the fight- flight- freeze response is, it is still activated in modern humans. It still has uses, even though we are far less likely to be preyed upon. It can help us power through a stressful event or have energy to accomplish beyond our usual performance. There is a downside, however, to the fight- flight- freeze response. For while it powers us up in some ways, it also damages tissues as it does so. It is rather like a turbo-charger on a car -- useful for short bursts of energy, but harmful if activated for long periods of time.

Thus, as we can see on the flow chart, the body needs a period of deep relaxation – the RELAXATION RESPONSE – in order to heal, to repair the tissue damage, and reduce the associated inflammation caused by the fight, flight, freeze response. In fact, this is the only route back to normal levels of autonomic arousal. That is, the body that is aroused in a fight- flight- freeze response can only return to normal after having had the profound relaxation of the relaxation response—slower pulse, lower blood pressure, sped up digestion, warm skin, and so on.

This is where the body-worker often enters the picture. Much body-work stimulates the relaxation response. Juhan in his magnificent text, *Job's Body* (2003) speaks to this and to the other important health benefits of body-work. Thus, body-work can play a very important role in stress management insofar as it triggers the relaxation response which, in turn, heals the bodily damage wrought by the fight- flight-freeze response.

This phenomenon is often encountered in the phenomenon we like to call "masked fatigue." Sometimes, when people have work done on the body that is relaxing, such as yoga, massage or a naprapathic treatment, they afterwards feel profoundly fatigued, to the point of exhaustion. Sometimes this fatigue is so deep that the individual can hardly stay awake and certainly finds it very hard to work. We understand this phenomenon as resulting from some individuals masking their fatigue and stress by "gutting it out," oftentimes by using stimulants like coffee or sugar to get them through the day. When the relaxation response is finally triggered by some effective body-work, it is as if the long withheld relaxation response takes over with a vengeance, and the individual lapses into deep fatigue. Sometimes this fatigue may linger on for days, even weeks. Inconvenient as the unmasking of the masked fatigue may be, it is ultimately an opportunity for the person to heal, to listen to his/her deep fatigue and perhaps to consider restructuring his life so as to build in the relaxation response more frequently so as to take better care of his body. This deep fatigue is perhaps linked to a weakened immune system (Daruna,2004) and chronic inflammation. Thus, the relaxation response should help strengthen both of these.

Many body-workers find themselves in the position of offering advice to their clients. Sometimes the advice may include exercise such as walking, swimming, stretching or weight-bearing.

If we look at Diagram 8 again, we can see that one route back to "normal levels" of arousal runs through substitute fight- flight- freeze activities. It is almost as if we can "trick" the fight- flight- freeze circuitry of the autonomic nervous system into "thinking" that we have in fact fought or run away or held stock still from a while. For example, if we go for a run or do some aerobics or swim, the autonomic nervous system receives input that seems to say, "All is well, you have run away or fought for your life." And after a while, one feels a deep sense of relaxation, one sleeps more deeply, and one's level of autonomic arousal returns to normal, having been healed by the body's excursion with the relaxation response (due to activation of the parasympathetic nervous system).

Body-workers often give "prescriptions" or advice regarding exercise—movement, stretching, weights, aerobics." These practitioners are well advised to bear in mind the relationship such activity has to the stress cycle. Perhaps these prescriptions will uncover masked fatigue or repressed memories. Perhaps the realignment of the autonomic nervous system will lead to a reduction of disorders related to stress, be they chronic or acute.

Clive Hazell PhD and Rosalinda Perez D.N.

Patterns of Response to Stress and its Relationship to Body Work

Now that we have reasonably established that body-workers will frequently encounter bodily and emotional manifestations of people's responses to trauma and stress, it seems worthwhile to examine some of the theories about human's response to these so the body-worker will be better prepared to help her/his patients. Each of the models offers some valuable insights.

Hans Selye (1978) offers the classic model of the organism's response to life stresses. Diagram 9 below illustrates his scheme.

Diagram 9: Selye's General Adaptation Syndrome

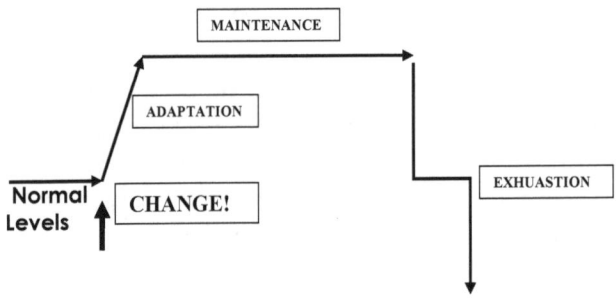

Selye's model shows a general pattern of physical response to stress. We start with levels of bodily arousal (e.g. blood pressure, adrenalin, pulse) at or near normal levels. Then a stress is introduced that calls upon the body to change. It does so by activating the fight-flight- freeze response, along with any other changes that are needed to adapt. The body then maintains its response to the change for as long as it can. Eventually, however, it gives way and the adaptive response exhausts.

While this is a physiologically based model, we believe it has many applications in the psychological realm. A trauma is visited upon us and we may attempt to adapt to it through an array of defensive maneuvers. We may use denial, repression, displacement, projection or any of the multiple forms of energy-consuming self protective "mind games" to adjust. We maintain these defense mechanisms for as long as we can, but, just as we can only stand on one leg for so long, so we can only rely on these self- protective maneuvers for so long. They exhaust and the individual starts to develop symptoms related to this exhaustion. Perhaps her sleep becomes disturbed or she feels depressed or anxious or loses the ability to concentrate. Often, at this point enough time has passed so that neither the individual nor those related to him or her connect these symptoms to the original stressor. All too often the symptoms are treated as if they were a mysterious disease, not as a delayed and rational response to an earlier trauma. For example, perhaps some cases of "chronic fatigue syndrome" can be understood as emanating from the "exhaustion" phase of the General Adaptation Syndrome.

Recognizing Burnout

Cherniss (1980) offers a very helpful model of the phenomenon of burnout in individuals working in high stress positions. Particularly helpful are the many signs and symptoms of burnout that we might not otherwise recognize as such. Figure 10 below represents aspects of the model Cherniss presents.

Diagram 10: Cherniss' Stages in the Burnout Process

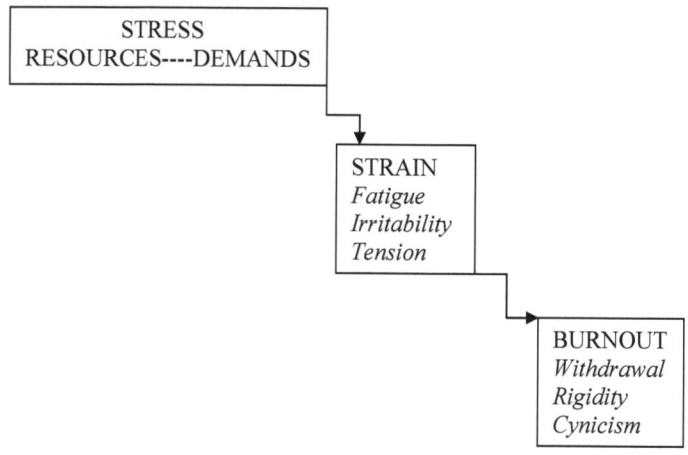

As we can see in this stage model of burnout, under normal operating conditions we are under stress, where the demands we face are reasonably balanced with an adequate amount of resources to meet those demands. We are confronted, in other words, with problems and challenges but we have enough time, money, materials and assistance to meet those challenges. This might also be called "eustress," that is, positive stress, or what Cziksentzmihalyi (2008) calls "flow" where we are challenged just enough to cause us to grow, to feel alive, even perhaps wonderful.

However, if the equation becomes unbalanced and demands outstrip resources, we enter into a condition of strain which is no longer productive and is evidenced by signs of fatigue, irritability and tension. Often individuals adjust to these as chronic unavoidable conditions of life, and often these can develop into significant physical complaints. Strain, however, is not the end of the story, for if it goes on for too long, it can develop into the condition of burnout. In this state, it is as if the individual has retired into a self-protective shell of withdrawal, rigidity and cynicism. People who are burned out avoid contact, especially emotional contact, are unwilling to change and often have given up on any ideals they may have had when first entering the profession to which they belong. Unfortunately, these very traits tend to ward off many attempts made by others to assist. In addition, burnout is often accompanied by a litany of physical complaints (somatization disorders). It is important for the body-worker to be aware that many physical complaints they encounter may have some or even much of their origin in the workplace environment of their patients. Sometimes physical health can be improved when individuals make adjustments in their work situation.

Loss, Grief, Mourning and the Body

Of course, one of the most painful and disruptive stresses humans must face is that of loss. Loss comes in many guises: loss of a loved one, of a job, of functionality, of an ideal of one's self worth, of an illusion. Many times these losses will somatize, that is, they will manifest as not only psychological, but also as physiological phenomena. Sometimes the physical reaction will be a result of the stress of the situation and will emanate from the changes in the autonomic nervous system. Sometimes, as seems to be the case in the next vignette, there are other more symbolic psychological responses to the loss, psychological responses that "capture" the feelings and thoughts associated with the loss in the person's body.

Case Vignette: Bodily pain as a result of complicated mourning.

Lail was a 64-year-old woman who came to the clinic complaining of chronic lower back pain and leg pain. As is so often the case, as the physical work was being done she started to talk about her life. She had lost her husband suddenly due to a heart attack some four years ago. Interestingly, he had pain in exactly the same leg. Every time Lail visits the clinic she cries about the loss of her husband, reminisces over his many good qualities and the times they spent together. She reports that she feels better after each session. The clinician simply does her work, empathically listens to her in an encouraging way, and resonates with her grief when she cries. After a few sessions Lail reveals that she also lost her mother at the age of eighteen months. Although she does not seem to evince emotional pain over this, the therapist notes to herself that this must have been traumatic for the toddler (who had recently discovered the use of her legs) and that this loss may have been activated upon the sudden loss of her husband.

Lail illustrates concepts from Freud's early paper, "Mourning and Melancholia," (1915). In it, he argues that "normal" mourning goes through several stages of grief, ending up with the bereaved person accepting the loss of the dead person. His grief lifts and he is able to move on with his life. However, there are numerous factors that can complicate the mourning process. If the loss is sudden and the ego is unprepared for the loss, or if there are lots of mixed feelings for the dead person, or feelings of guilt, the mourning gets derailed and the bereaved, instead of letting the person go and holding on to memories, identifies with the departed. He in some way becomes the departed person, as if to deny he has in fact gone. This, according to Freud, can result in melancholia, and other related symptoms. Perhaps Lail, who lost her husband unexpectedly, is suffering from a bodily form of derailed mourning. She seems to have incorporated her lost husband's pain in his legs. Interestingly (and as is predicted by Freudian theory) as she speaks of his loss and experiences the grief (especially with another as a witness to her loss and pain) so the incorporation subsides, and is replaced by memories. In the case of Lail, we see how carefully synthesized body-work and empathy can help the patient literally, "get back on her feet."

Lail's case brings us to the question, "What is to be expected if one goes through the mourning process in a healthy way? What happens if one does not get derailed in the mourning process? How might these processes show up in bodywork?" Elizabeth Kubler-Ross (1993) and Verena Kast (1993) provide us with templates that can be of help in charting that process. These templates should not be used by the clinician or anyone, for that matter, in a lockstep fashion. They are probably best used as a set of guidelines to help the individual sensitize and prepare themselves for whatever the bereaved person needs to accomplish at that given stage and to facilitate his/her working it through. Other psychologists also argue that the scheme can be worked through in other orders than that presented by Kubler-Ross.

Diagram 11 gives a diagrammatic representation of Kubler-Ross's well-known scheme.

Diagram 11: Kubler Ross's Model of the Mourning Process

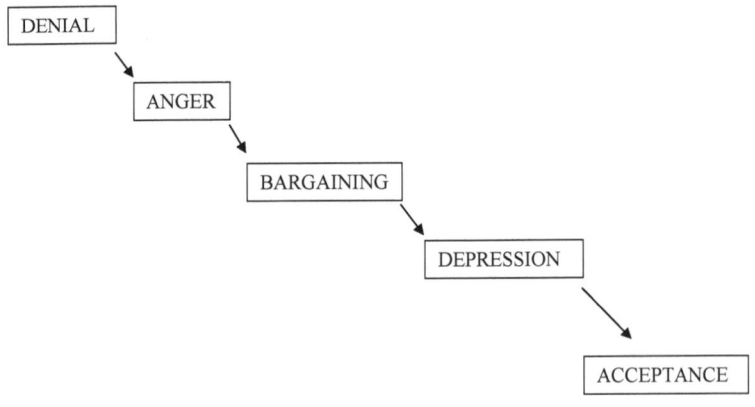

(1969, "Death and Dying, New York, Macmillan)

The first response of the individual when they are confronted with a terminal illness (or as we believe with any other significant loss) is that of denial. "I do not believe it!" seems to be the classic initial response. Eventually this denial gives way and the person, in facing the reality of his situation becomes angry, and this anger can be directed at others or himself, often at the very people trying to help him the most. The anger then fades and the person attempts to make some sort of a deal; perhaps to gain more time, or to get a cure or reverse his plight. When these attempts fail, the person seems to fall into a depression. They become demoralized and despondent. They lose interest in many things and feel miserable and despairing; all hope seems to have gone. Ultimately this depression gives way to a sense of acceptance as the person adjusts to his new situation and the loss he confronts. It is a peaceful but realistic state of mind that the person is in at this stage, as if he has come to terms with his situation.

Verena Kast provides us with a slightly different take from Kubler Ross. Her approach is based on Jungian psychology. It does not contradict Kubler-Ross's theory. It offers a different and useful perspective. Diagram 12 below gives a diagrammatic representation of her scheme.

Diagram 12: Schematic of Kast's "A Time to Mourn"

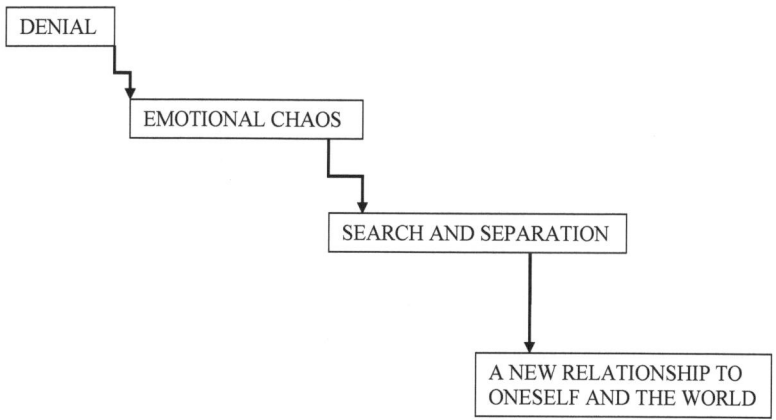

As we can see, Kast's model has the individual reacting to loss initially with denial, an unwillingness to accept the reality of the situation, as if the mind is numbing itself to pain by cutting off full awareness of the event. This gives way to emotional chaos, where all of the painful feelings of grief seem to visit the person, often unexpectedly, causing terrible disruption in his emotional life and behavior. This is then followed by search and separation, where the person makes attempts to regain contact with the person (or thing) that has been lost. Sometimes this attempt is behavioral, where the person will attempt to reinstate that which was lost by doing what he used to do with the person, or by being like the person in some way. Sometimes the attempt at recovering that which was lost takes place during dreams where the individual has vivid dreams that the person they lost is alive and well. Gradually, these attempts are seen as hopeless, the search ends and the person establishes a new relationship to himself and the world. He can go on as a new person; he can start the next chapter of his life.

The reason we present these models of the mourning process is that body-workers will often work with individuals who are actively working through the mourning process or who have somehow been derailed in the process. Body-work can often activate a dormant unworked mourning process. The body-worker thus should be prepared for the psychological side of the patient's recovery as it accompanies the physical recovery. These models perhaps will sensitize the body-worker to some of the issues they might encounter.

CHAPTER 11

Sexuality and Body Work

Sexual responsiveness obviously involves the body. Body-work, if successful, will probably help the patient's sexual functioning, perhaps by increasing range of motion, by reducing pain or by increasing the connection with the body and the overall sense of "aliveness." It is also quite likely that from time to time body-work will cause sexual arousal in the patient. This will be obviously more visible with males than females, but in either case the body-worker will need to have done some serious thinking about his own relationship to his body and about his own sexuality before he embarks on a career that involves touching the bodies of others, especially in contexts that encourage regression such as lying down and being cared for.

The following case vignette gives an example of the way in which an intervention that is technically valid may be misinterpreted by the patient, thus bringing an unnecessary early end to treatment.

Case example: The Psoas and Sexuality

A female naprapath had been seeing a male patient, age 32, for several visits. She had been working on his lower back and he mentioned that his discomfort had eased considerably. Much of his pain came from strains and stresses involved in his work. Perhaps encouraged by this, the male patient mentioned he also had pain in his shoulders and upper back. The naprapath worked with these areas and the patient, as before, reported relief. As this happened, the patient mentioned that the pain in his lower back had returned. At this the naprapath worked on the iliopsoas, the long muscle running through the pelvis from the thoracic vertebrae to the thigh. There was considerable tension in this muscle and the patient reported considerable relief and relaxation as he left. However, he never returned and the naprapath believed that his not returning had something to do with her working on his psoas.

Although we cannot be sure, this hypothesis is quite plausible. Some of her colleagues wondered if the client terminated because of embarrassing sexual feelings he may have felt when having his psoas palpated. After some discussion, they felt that it was most likely the patient had not felt sexually stimulated so much as he had felt vulnerable. This idea is consistent with bioenergetic theory. The pelvis is often (even usually) an area of deep vulnerability, where many tender emotions can be "locked up." Body-work in these areas can stir up these feelings, and if the patient is unprepared for them, they may become flooded with emotion or sense that deep and powerful emotions are surfacing, and decide to distance themselves from the situation.

In retrospect, perhaps it would have been advisable for the naprapath to have discussed in a tactful, non-alarmist way these ideas with the patient who at least would be psychologically prepared for any emotional responses he might have had to work in the pelvic area. The next case is similar in the physical problem that is presented. The interaction between the body-worker and the patient, however, leads to a more positive outcome.

Mention the psoas, that large deep muscle extending all the way from the thoracic spine to the femur through the pelvis to a group of body-workers and you almost certainly will get some strong reactions. Entire books have been written on this muscle and its psychological importance (Koch, 1997). Alexander Lowen also places it in pride of place as a container of emotional issues. It is often connected with issues related to the spine, one's "backbone." It is also connected to one's sexuality, since it passes through the pelvis and controls much of its motility. In addition, it affects one's posture, one's "standing." Many body-workers, perhaps because of the location of the *psoas* and its saturation with emotional meaning, simply learn to avoid work with it. In addition, many patients will resist working with it. Working in that region, often in the area of the pelvis, is experienced with great vulnerability. Often simply to touch this muscle is very painful since it has been so long ignored and is often chronically inflamed. The following vignette gives an example of this resistance and one naprapath's response.

Case Vignette: "David Beckham"

David was a thirty- year-old male, very thin and an aficionado of the beautiful game, soccer. David Beckham was his hero. He played frequently, as frequently as he could given his debilitating and chronic back spasms. He was thin and his body was tense throughout, evidencing his frequent workouts with little stretching and a driven, almost obsessive streak in his personality. The naprapath formed the opinion that the problem lay in a tightly contracted psoas that was mis-aligning the spine, pelvis and femur and creating a great deal of compression in the lumbar region, the area of his pain. After some more peripheral work, with the quadriceps, calves and ileo-tibial band, she gave warning that she was about to make some contact with the psoas. This warning is often recognized as important so as to prepare the patient for the stress of this type of bodily intervention. In addition, work with the psoas should start out very slowly, usually with simple touch, so as not to cause the patient to mobilize their defenses too radically and also in recognition of the fact that for many (perhaps most) people the psoas is very, very tender. The naprapath made long and sensitive attempts to engage therapeutic contact with the psoas, but to no avail. The patient seemed to fight tooth and nail, remaining closed off, not letting the naprapath in to the deeper zones where the problem seemed to be. At this point the naprapath decided to make a confrontation. She said, "You are not letting me in, and that is O.K. But if you do not let me in, I cannot help you. I know that much of why you are keeping me out is because it is sensitive, but I also think that some of it is emotional. When you are ready to face these emotions, you will let me in, and then you will not have to keep on coming back to me forever. I am not trying to pressure you. I am simply framing a decision that I think you have to make."

Bit by bit, the patient was able to allow the naprapath deeper and deeper access to the psoas and his chronic back problem did ease. He never shared the emotional side of his bodily issues with the naprapath. Perhaps this was done elsewhere, with his girlfriend, friends, or in solitary contemplation. Perhaps it happened unconsciously; perhaps not at all. Sometimes the body-worker is used as a container and organizer of emotional responses from the patient, sometimes not.

Probably first among the concerns of body-workers is to become comfortable with sexual responsiveness in such a way that they can discriminate between sexual arousal in patients that is basically just the body "doing its thing" and sexual arousal that is more of a "come on." Massage therapists and body-workers who use the technique of rocking will notice that it often will cause an erection in men, but that this erection is simply the natural response of the body in this form of motion. Most patients will probably have this understanding, too. Other patients, however may experience this with much anxiety and feel guilty and ashamed, perhaps not returning for treatment. Still others may respond with expectations that the body-worker gratify their sexual needs. At this point of course, the body-worker will be expected to be comfortable enough about his personal and professional boundaries to state that that is not what he is there to do.

Sometimes the "come on's" are blunt and direct, such as when a patient, after having a massage that involved elbow palpation of the *gluteus maximus* asked the therapist to "finish me off." The therapist was surprised by the request and pointed out that the establishment they were in was hardly the kind of place for that and, while he was willing to continue work as a massage therapist, there would be no sexual interaction whatever.

Sometimes, the "propositions" are more subtle, perhaps even slick, as when a client is very charming and polite but has little "accidents" of a revealing and suggestive nature. Nothing is said, but the intention is clear and the air is thick with suggestion. These situations can be more uncomfortable than the direct requests.

The sexualization of the body-work can occur even if the therapist is very professional in his demeanor and very careful that where he touches and how he touches is not interpretable as titillating or seductive. On the other hand, we believe that it is possible for the therapist to be unaware of the nature of his touch, so careful supervision is required in this area.

Further, certain personality types and those with histories of sexual abuse might be more prone to sexualize the body-work experience than others. When we examine the histories of patients who are victims of sexual contact with their psychotherapists, we find that those with histories of sexual abuse are very over-represented.

Sometimes the sexuality is coated in romance and the patient will fall in love. Josef Breuer, who was Freud's early colleague, is reputed to have left the field of psychoanalysis early because the 'positive transferences' of his female patients falling in love with him was a bit too much to bear. Body-work, as we have repeatedly pointed out, is extremely regressive. It stimulates powerful transferences. Sometimes these take the form of the patient falling in love or wanting to have sexual relationships with the therapist. It is sometimes as if the patient, starved of maternal love, has finally found that perfect person and has decided he will have her forever and for always.

Sometimes people sexualize the experience because sexuality is less anxiety producing than what is being stimulated by the body-work. For example, if the body-work is stimulating an intense fear or rage, the person might unconsciously decide to feel sexy as a more bearable alternative, as a way of taking her mind off these troubling thoughts.

In addition, body-work, as noted at the outset, can lead to improvements in one's sex life. This is wonderful; however, it can also lead to problems. Lowen points out and we have seen elsewhere in this book how "pleasure anxiety" can be a stumbling block. Also, such increases in sexual aliveness can put stress on marital relationships, for example, where the partners have become habituated to a certain level of sexual desire and activity. This increased aliveness goes back into the family and will cause changes, positive we hope, but changes, nonetheless of which the therapist should be aware.

Sexual Trauma and the Body

Sexual assault, trauma and molestation present a special set of responses that the body-worker will encounter. Sutherlin and Schierl (1970) discovered an interestingly similar pattern amongst a sample of women who had been raped. Diagram 13, below shows the three phases they identified.

Diagram 13: Patterns of Response Amongst Women Victims of Rape

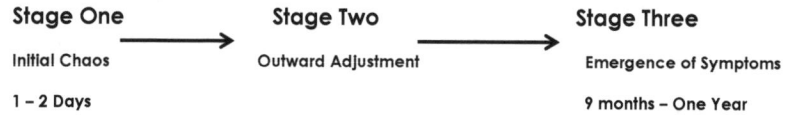

Stage One	Stage Two	Stage Three
Initial Chaos	Outward Adjustment	Emergence of Symptoms
1 – 2 Days		9 months – One Year

The parallels between this psychological pattern and Selye's model are clear. The individual, after going through a period of disorientation in response to the trauma, seems to adjust, to "get over" the shock and go back to "life as usual." This pattern is maintained for as long as possible. In their study, this turned out to be nine months, but our clinical impression is that there is considerable variability in this period. We have colleagues who have encountered memories of sexual trauma "breaking through" to the surface after fifty years of repression. Eventually this outward adjustment gives way and the person becomes symptomatic. Often these symptoms will not be seen as connected to the original trauma. Often too, these symptoms will take on a physical form; they will be somatoform and the individual will visit a body-worker. Let us hope that the body-worker has some awareness of the human response to stress, because this awareness will become an important part of the treatment program.

Introducing touch into the treatment of a person who has been physically or sexually abused.

Most psychological counselors are all too well aware that the incidence of sexual and physical abuse is much higher in the general population that is generally supposed. This is especially true amongst women, where many studies point to about one in five adult women having been victims of sexual abuse at some point during their lives. Clearly all the material in this book will potentially apply to this group of patients. In addition, it will be of use for the body-worker to be aware of some ideas and techniques that may help the individual gain increased comfort with the touching that body-work involves.

First, it is important to note that an individual may be unaware of her discomfort at being touched or, more frequently, at being touched in certain areas or in certain ways, until it actually happens. Several women in our practices, for example, evinced great surprise at their strong emotional reactions of fear, sadness or anger when their husbands or boyfriends unexpectedly tickled them or hugged them from behind. Not only were these clients surprised, they also did not immediately connect their strong, emotional responses to past sexual or physical abuse. It would sometimes take several weeks for this painful realization to take place.

This would mean that it is possible for a patient to start treatment with a body-worker and to suddenly and unexpectedly have intense emotional responses to certain kinds of touch or touch itself. We predict that, while the gender of the participants may often play a role, it is not always going to be "locked in." For example, a woman who has been abused by a man could have strong reactions to touch, even though the body-worker is a woman. The reason for this prediction is that body-work, especially when it involves lying down, can be extremely regressive (almost hypnotic), regressive in such a way that gender is not registered with much, if any, clarity. Also, issues pertaining to gender can often become confused in cases of sexual abuse, and the concept of gender can easily slip into the background of perception, or be eclipsed by more potent and pressing concerns, such as physical pain or one's safety.

When one has a client who wishes to do body-work but finds they have strong emotional responses to touch that "get in the way," perhaps some straightforward ideas from behavioristic psychology could work. The three ideas are *successive approximation, positive reinforcement and densitization.*

Successive approximation means that we approach the behavioral goal one baby step at a time. We start from wherever we are at the beginning, which might, in this case, mean that the patient is willing to sit in a room with you and discuss body-work and move, slowly but surely, up an anxiety gradient, rewarding (positively reinforcing) each step of the way until the final goal is reached. The rewards usually do not have to be complex. Simple verbal encouragement goes a long way.

As the client moves up a notch, takes the next step and her anxiety increases, she is encouraged to use previously learned relaxation procedures, such as deep, slow breathing, focusing, imaging or any type of a whole litany of techniques that can relax. Thus the client gradually expands her realm of relaxed behavior to include ultimately the target set of behaviors and body-work can proceed.

A sample hierarchy of successive approximations for a client anxious about touch might be:

STEPS:
1. Sit in the room and discuss background.

2. Sit in the room and observe film of body-work.

3. Sit in room and observe live body-work being performed on another person.

4. Have body-worker work on parts of the body that are very easy to touch.

5. Same as step four, but include one more area of a bit more difficulty (still clothed).

6. Repeat step 5.

7. Return to step 4, but unclothed.

8. Repeat step 5 until workable level of contact is reached.

It is important to recall that at each step the client will be likely to experience an upsurge in anxiety and will need time to relax and to process the feelings they are having in relation to the increased bodily contact. At times, this process may move quite smoothly and the body-worker will have the clear feeling that she is functioning in the role of a body-worker, and simply helping the patient get to a point where she can conformably engage in body-work. In other words, she will not feel like she is being a clinical psychologist. At other times, however, the body-worker will have the impression that she is at the edge of her professional training and that the client she is working with is in need of professional counseling. At that point, the body-worker should make a referral (unless they themselves are a licensed psychologist, counselor, psychotherapist or mental health professional).

This case illustrates the delicacy of working with patients who have been sexually traumatized, and that areas other than the pelvic zone can be associated with memories of trauma and abuse.

Case Vignette: Densitization:

Charles was a man in his 40's who had been sexually abused when he was a child. He was gay and HIV positive. A large, though not obese man, he was shy and soft-spoken. He came to the massage therapist with the explicit purpose of "desensitizing myself to men's touch".

The first therapy involved some gentle myofascial work and Charles responded positively, stating that he felt "empowered" and "healthy." In the next session, the therapist worked behind the upper back and with the collarbones to help "thoracic outlet," holding the position for some thirty seconds. At this, Charles reported "something....very upset." He held his breath, started quivering and tears started to flow, even though the pressure was minimal, and actually more supportive. The therapist asked, "Do you need me to stop?" and he slowly removed his hands. Gradually, Charles was able to speak. "It's reminding me of when I was controlled and attacked. It's taking me back. I feel scared." The therapist replied, "No problem. Let me know how you feel. Perhaps I could work on the top of your head?" And so the therapist continued work on the top of Charles' head. Charles kept his eyes open, as if to stay anchored in the present and not have any more flashbacks. In addition, he engaged the therapist in small talk. The session ended and Charles came back for two more visits a month or so later. These sessions did not involve such emotional responses.

D. Winnicott (1960), R, D, Laing (1969) and Alexander Lowen (2005) have written extensively on the phenomenon of disembodiment, pointing out that when people are traumatized, they commonly lose contact with their bodies, with concomitant sensations of numbness, estrangement and alienation. This can have disastrous results on the individuals biopsychosocial well being. Body-work provides a wonderful vehicle for helping individuals get back in touch with the reality of their bodies. As this section and much of this book shows, this process is not an easy one, but it can be a very effective one. We believe it is unfortunate that body-work is not given more pride of place in the treatment of trauma.

SECTION IV: INTERPERSONAL RELATIONS AND THE PRACTICE OF BODY WORK

In this section, we shift the focus again. Here we examine some ways in which interpersonal relationships can enter into the practice of body-work. First, we will examine some fairly common categories of personality types and look at some of the ways these different types might influence the treatment relationship. Then, we will examine the cluster of phenomena that are called "somatoform disorders" in the "Diagnostic and Statistical Manual" (1994) and finally we will look at some of the more "difficult" personality types one might encounter as a body-worker (the so-called "personality disorders") and how one might understand and work with them profitably.

CHAPTER 12

Psychological Type and the Practice of Body-Work

In this section we examine the ways in which different personality types interact in the treatment situation. How does a warm-hearted extraverted doctor interact with a shy introverted patient? What are the plusses and minuses of being more spontaneous, of, "letting things happen", versus approaching life with a plan. To examine these questions, we will use Carl Gustav Jung's theory of psychological types (1971). It is a "user-friendly" and non pejorative exploration of different personality styles. You can get a copy of the Myers Briggs type Inventory (MBTI) to find out your personality type, from a wide array of online sources, as well as from professional counselors. We also highly recommend consultation of the book, "Gifts Differing," (Myers, J., 1995).

For purely illustrative purposes, we have constructed a short questionnaire below to give you a quick beginning idea of the constructs involved and to get you started thinking about these dimensions and how they might affect your practice. Warning: This instrument has not been statistically validated in any way. If you want to find out your psychological type from the validated version of the MBTI, we recommend you check with a licensed counselor or psychologist.

QUICK TEST OF TYPE

Rate the statements below from 1 to 5 where:

5 means the statement is "Very like me"
4 means the statement is "Like me"
3 indicates that the statement is "Neither like me nor unlike me."
2 indicates that the statement is "Unlike me"
1 indicates that the statement is "Very unlike me"

1. __I like meeting new people.
2. __I like being on my own.
3. __I like to deal with the present.
4. __I like to imagine possibilities.
5. __I trust logic.
6. __I follow my feelings.
7. __I enjoy spontaneity.
8. __I prefer my day to be planned.
9. __I get energy from other people.
10. __I get energy from within myself.
11. __I like practical things.
12. __I like possibilities.
13. __I like theories and reasoning.
14. __I like to follow my heart.
15. __I like change.
16. __I like order.
17. __I like starting conversations.
18. __I enjoy my time apart from others.
19. __I am detail-minded.
20. __I look for the big patterns.
21. __I like to follow my head, my reasoning.
22. __I trust my feelings.
23. __I like doing things on the spur of the moment.
24. __I like doing things on time.
25. __I enjoy being with people.
26. __Solitude is precious to me.
27. __I like routine.

28. __I like fantasy.
29. __Reason leads to the best decisions.
30. __Emotions guide my behavior.
31. __I like to let things happen.
32. __I like to plan ahead.
33. __I enjoy being in a group.
34. __I like to work alone.
35. __I like learning practical things.
36. __I like dreaming.
37. __I enjoy analyzing problems.
38. __I respond first to problems with my feelings.
39. __I like to just "hang out" and see what comes up.
40. __I like to schedule my time.

Scoring: Add the numbers you entered for each item and total across to give yourself a score out of twenty for each of the eight dimensions below. The higher your score, the more you fit the typology. (Bear in mind that the instrument has not been validated statistically. It is just to to give you an initial "feel" for the theory.)

	Item scores	Total
Extraversion:	1__, 9__, 17__, 25__, 33__	E_____
Introversion:	2__, 10__, 18__, 26__, 34__	I_____
Sensing:	3__, 11__, 19__, 27__, 35__	S_____
Intuition:	4__, 12__, 20__, 28__, 36__	N_____
Thinking:	5__, 13__, 21__, 29__, 37__	T_____
Feeling:	6__, 14__, 22__, 30__, 38__	F_____
Perceiving:	7__, 15__, 23__, 31__, 39__	P_____
Judging:	8__, 16__, 24__, 32__, 40__	J_____

People do have individual styles and these can be interestingly captured on an instrument such as the MBTI. Many things that go on in the practice of body-work can be explained, at least in part, by using the concepts, categories and insights from the MBTI. Indeed, since the MBTI itself is based on the work, *Psychological Types* by C. G. Jung, a wide array of further interpretive avenues and lines of thought are opened up.

In this section, therefore, we will examine the four pairs of the basic dimensions of the typology, explore how these might help explain some dynamics of families, and further, examine how different psychological types might manifest themselves in doctor-patient interactions.

One determines one's type by seeing where one lies on four pairs of opposites, as shown below: (add the item scores and compare them pairwise, the larger one is one's type.)

Extraversion (E)...........Introversion (I)
Sensing (S).............Intuition (N)
Thinking (T).........Feeling (F)
Judging (J).............Perceiving (P)

Note that if the spread between the scores, say E and I is large, say more than ten points, this indicates possibly a strong preference for one way of o[operating over another. If they are close, say within a few points of each other, it may indicate that you can switch styles a bit more easily.

Extraversion - Introversion

This dimension has to do with the basic orientation of the personality. The extrovert directs his/her attention toward the outside world and the introvert directs his/her attention toward the inner world. Usually, but not always, the extrovert is outgoing and the introvert is more retiring. Jung felt that extroverts and introverts would often marry. Two married extroverts might compete for "airspace" while two introverts might drift apart. Furthermore, we often marry someone who is our opposite in terms of type so as to stimulate our growth, our self completion. Extroverts tend to reach out to other people for "energy" while introverts tend to look inside themselves when they need a boost.

Are you more extroverted or introverted?

Why do you say this?

Do you find yourself more attracted to introverts or extroverts? Why?

How does your type (E or I) affect practice?

<u>Sensing - Intuition</u>

This dimension of Jung's typology has much to do with what types of information we regard as valid. Sensing types trust their senses (touch, sight, sound, smell, taste). They rely heavily on sensory data and are thus very practical and often detail minded. Intuitive types, on the other hand, rely on imagination and are fascinated by possibility, by conjecture. They tend, therefore, to be more like "dreamers" or even visionaries. Intuitives might forget to "read the small print" or to take care of everyday chores, and they may prefer new beginnings to mundane chores. Sensing types, however, may not "see the forest for the trees" and get lost in details. In this way, these two types need each other and profit from collaboration.

Do you consider yourself more "sensing" or "intuitive," in the sense used by Jung? Why?

What are the consequences of this personal orientation (S or N)...?

a. in your practice?

b. in your career?

Thinking - Feeling

This dimension, to simplify somewhat, has to do with the extent to which a person is ruled by logic (their "head") or by human values and feelings (their "heart"). The thinking type of person will face moral dilemmas, make decisions and comport himself based on logic. The feeling person will see this as rather cold and unemotional, uncaring and diffident. Oftentimes, couples or parents and children will get involved in arguments over decisions that emanate from the different approaches of thinking and feeling. The thinking type may espouse a disciplinary system based on logic, while the feeling type may find such an intellectual approach to human relations very unsatisfactory and alien.

Do you think you are more of a thinking or a feeling type?

Give an example to illustrate how you are like this.

How do you like to argue...with logic (thinking) or with human values (feeling)?

How does your preference (T or F) affect your practice?

Judging and Perceiving

The "judging" type of person prefers an ordered, predictable life; they plan and organize, they like to show up on time and keep to a schedule. The "perceiving" type, on the other hand, prefers spontaneity; they like to "hang out," to just let things happen; they might not mind showing up late or when plans go awry; they might even enjoy some chaos.

Again, these individual differences could show up in family life. One member could be "judging" (note: not judgmental) and like life to be orderly and tidy. Another member may be "perceiving" and like a more free-wheeling lifestyle. It takes little to imagine the conflicts that might emerge. "Can't you ever be on time?" exclaims one. "Can't you just relax and let things happen, go with the flow?" responds the other.

Do you consider yourself more "judging" or "perceiving"? Why?

How does this affect your practice?

Give an example to illustrate your assessment.

Psychological Type and Conflict

Following is a table of some typical conflicts between types. Some conflicts can be usefully understood as conflicts based on type.

Extroverts will often say of introverts:
- You're not expressive enough.
- Why do I have to keep the conversation going?
- Why don't you tell me how you feel?

Introverts will often say to extroverts:
- Can we just be quiet for a while?
- Stop pressuring me to open up.
- Why do we have to communicate?

Sensing types will often say to intuitives:
- Keep your feet on the ground!
- Why can't you be more practical?
- I need to <u>see</u> how it is done.

Intuitives will often say to sensing types:
- Why do you have to be so practical?
- Can't we dream and imagine?
- There's more to things than meets the eye.

Feeling types will often say to thinking types:
- You're so cool and aloof.
- Not everything is logical, you know.
- But what do you <u>feel</u>?

Thinking types will often say to feeling types:
- You should think things through, and not be lead by your heart.
- I have feelings too, you know.
- Your feelings aren't the best guide.

Judging types might say to perceiving types:
- Could you get things done on time?
- Will you make a plan, please?

- We need to get this organized.

Perceiving types might say to judging types:
- Can we just "hang out" and see what happens?
- Can you be more spontaneous?
- Let's forget the plan!

Alternatively, opposite types can be of great help to one another, both immediately and in that each can stimulate and challenge the growth of the other.

How the types can help one another: The Usefulness of Opposites

The extrovert needs the introvert to:
- explore the inner world
- interpret dreams
- learn how to be alone and introspect.

The introvert needs the extrovert to:
- connect with the outer world
- join the group or the crowd
- have fun with others, to communicate.

The intuitive needs the sensing type to:
- be practical
- read the contract
- make the day-to-day things work.

The sensing needs the intuitive to:
- dream of the future
- inspire
- open up possibilities.

The thinking type needs the feeling type to:
- help him/her understand others' hearts, to be warm-hearted
- persuade others
- make others feel wanted and important.

The feeling type needs the thinking type to:
- analyze
- finally make a decision
- keep a cool head.

The judging type needs the perceiving type to:
- have surprises
- have new experiences
- relax and be spontaneous.

The perceiving type needs the judging type to:
- get organized
- save time
- realize goals.

These lists are just beginnings. We encourage you to read further. There is a bibliography at the end of this book on several topics, including the MBTI.

Case Examples

To assist you in connecting this theory of personality types, the following activity asks you to identify three features of the doctor-patient relationship that would be helpful and three that would be potentially troublesome in the following doctor/patient pairings. Suggested answers are at the end of the section.

Pairing 1 :

Dr. A.   **Pt. Y**
ENFP   **ISTJ**

Three benefits of this pairing of types :

1.

2.

3.

Three potential difficulties arising from this pairing :

1.

2.

3.

Pairing Two :

Dr. B.   **Pt. Z**
ESTJ   **INFP**

Three positive features arising from this pairing.

1.

2.

3.

Three potential tensions arising from this pairing.

1.

2.

3.

Pairing three:

Dr. C.   **Pt. X**
INTJ   **ESFP**

Three potential plusses of this pairing.

1.

2.

3.

Three potential tensions in this relationship.

1.

2.

3.

Suggested Answers:

Pairing One: Dr. ESTJ and ISTJ patient.

Among the difficulties this pairing might find we could include the following: The doctor might be very much a "slap you on the back" type and this could overwhelm the shy introverted patient who might need a bit more time to come out of his or her shell. They are both thinking types and like organization. This, although it could be a plus, might cause them to overlook some of the important emotional issues in their healing relationship. The doctor may think that if everything has been managed well, then the problem is solved. They are both sensing types who will rely on their sensory impressions to evaluate situations and will regard with suspicion ideas that are intuitive, even though they may be useful ones. The doctor, being an extrovert, may have more of a tendency to spread him or herself around more than the patient, so even though as an STJ, he or she should keep him/herself organized, he/she probably finds him/herself being a bit stressed out at times. This doctor will tend to feel comfortable in a group situation and in starting a relationship, while the patient will probably take a little more time to warm up. Both will tend to prefer a structured treatment program or process, and may thus shy away from more ambiguous situations or untested pathways.

Pairing Two: Dr. ESTJ and Patient INFP

Here again, we have an extroverted doctor and an introverted patient, so all that was said above about this pairing applies here. With this relationship, however, more difficulties could arise, because the other three functions are opposed. The doctor will tend to be very practical and down to earth, which could, of course help the patient appreciate the here and now reality of his/her situation, which he/she, as an intuitive, might overlook. On the other hand, the doctor may not listen to the patient's intuitive thoughts and ideas and these could be useful in gathering ideas as to what is going on in the life of the patient and in establishing emotional contact. The doctor is a thinking type and the patient is a feeling type. The doctor, therefore will tend to think that if the problem has been solved logically, the problem has indeed been solved. The patient, however, will not be happy until some emotional resolution has also been reached. The patient, also will tend to form more of an emotional connection with the doctor (as opposed to the thinking connection the previous patient will form with their doctor). This connection will not be immediately observable because of the privacy with which an introverted feeling type will tend to guard his/her emotions. The doctor may miss it, but this will be an error for very often this type can be quite emotionally sensitive, delicate, almost. They are found frequently in artistic professions, for example. The doctor, finally, is a J and will like to plan things out, while the patient is more spontaneous and may even be somewhat disorganized in his/her lifestyle. This could give rise to the obvious tensions around scheduling treatment, sticking to plans and keeping time arrangements.

Pairing three: Dr. INTJ and patient ESFP

Here we have an introverted, intuitive, thinking, judging doctor paired with an extroverted, sensing, feeling perceptive type. This "odd couple" is often the stuff of situation comedies, and just as in the stories, this relationship can, if its tensions are recognized and yoked to the tasks at hand, lead to a very interesting and creative relationship. If not, the results are less prepossessing. The doctor will tend to be retiring and the patient will be outgoing. The doctor will gain energy through isolated thinking and dreaming and the patient will desire emotional contact in the here and now. The doctor will be fascinated with theory and possibilities. The patient will be focused on the concrete practicalities and emotional nuances of the situation at hand. The doctor will aim for a plan, while the patient will aim for a freewheeling relational style of treatment. The doctor may be overwhelmed by the emotionality of the patient and the patient may find the doctor frustratingly remote and intellectualized. At times the doctor's remoteness may be experienced by the patient as calming; at others as uncaring and unempathic. The doctor may find the patient's lifestyle quite distressingly unorganized; while at other times he or she may find that it helps open him to other possibilities, other avenues of thought. There is a lot of potential energy in this relationship, as there are many oppositions. The patient will see boundaries as impediments to contact, while the doctor will see them as necessary for effective functioning. Perhaps the truth for this duo lies somewhere in between. This couple will perhaps function best to the extent that they are able to recognize this in their many areas of difference.

CHAPTER 13

Somatoform Disorders

The Diagnostic and Statistical Manual of the American Psychiatric association (DSM IV-R; 1994) provides a set of categories and a decision tree that provides a potentially useful framework for thinking about the bodily related psychological issues that may confront a clinician, be that clinician a psychologist, counselor, social worker, teacher, medical worker or body-worker. The categories are not simply cubby holes in which to place the patient's complaints. They do provide avenues for creatively and usefully thinking about patients and their underlying dynamics.

There are eleven different categories of somatoform disorders. We will not reproduce the decision tree from the DSM IV here but will describe the essential features of each type. We refer the reader to the DSM for further insight into the subtleties of the categories, especially if questions arise with regard to a given patient.

Following the descriptions we will provide several cases to give you practice on assessing patients and evaluating the utility of the scheme.

1. Psychological Factors Affecting Medical Condition

In this condition, the patient has an identifiable medical condition that is adversely affected by psychological factors. One could argue that every physical illness will be affected to some extent by psychological factors and that every illness will indeed generate psychological factors that affect the course of treatment and healing. This category is reserved for those individuals where the course of the illness is significantly worsened in one of several possible ways by psychological factors. For example a person suffering from depression may feel so hopeless that they see no point in the exercises the body-worker prescribes. An individual with passive-aggressive or dependent personality features may unconsciously resist treatment. In the first case, the cause may be unconscious resentment. In the latter, perhaps it is out of separation anxiety. Cognitive deficits may also be included in this category. An individual with diabetes and a learning disability, for example, may find it hard to understand the dynamics of the illness and the reasoning behind the dietary restrictions. In addition patients utilizing the defense mechanism of denial may not admit the significance of certain symptoms or test results.

Often, the medical practitioner or the body-worker does not have the training to be of direct help to the patient. Frequently, they might not even diagnose the interacting psychological condition, perhaps noting that it is frustrating to work with a certain patient or that they are not "compliant." Perhaps in these cases, in addition to empathy (which hardly ever fails), the body-worker may tactfully suggest some counseling or a support group to the patient.

2. **Factitious Disorder**

This condition involves the intentional feigning of a physical or psychological condition, often for purpose of assuming the role of a sick person. The patient only gets the "reward" of taking up the role of patient. There must be no other external incentive for having the illness such as economic gain, time off work, avoidance of a responsibility. If there are such gains for the patient then the condition is defined as "malingering" and the dynamics are significantly different.

This is the condition also known as "von Munchausen's syndrome." Often times one notices in patients displaying this condition that they have a history of medical procedures and a good knowledge of medical terminology. Frequently, they can be quite argumentative with practitioners and seem to derive a sense of specialness from their frequently "mysterious" illnesses.

Factitious disorder by proxy is when another person is presented as the patient. Often this involves a parent bringing in a child who has taken up the role of patient, all this in the absence of any external rewards for being sick. It is as if the parent gains some sense of satisfaction from taking up the role of the parent with a sick child. The child, by virtue of their dependence and suggestibility, often has been subtly convinced that they are indeed sick.

3. **Malingering**

Malingering is the intentional faking of symptoms so that the patient gains some other reward. This intentional deception may be activated in order to avoid legal responsibility, for economic gain, to avoid work, to avoid dangerous assignments or to obtain drugs. Often times the practitioner can be tipped off to the possibility of malingering when the patient's life situation seems to indicate that there would be distinct advantages to being "sick" at this point in time. Additionally there may be a marked discrepancy between the objective findings and the patient's complaints. The practitioner may also notice a lower level of compliance in the malingering patient. Malingering may be more common among persons with antisocial personality features, that is, persons who seem to lack a sense of concern for others while displaying a very egocentric attitude towards life.

Malingering is different from factitious disorder insofar as there is a clear external incentive to be in the sick role. This is not the case with factitious disorder. Malingering is different from conversion disorder and other somatoform disorders insofar as the symptoms are intentionally, consciously created with a clear view to an end. This is not the case in the other disorders, where treatment techniques involving the unconscious might work.

4. **Somatization Disorder**

This disorder, which was previously known as Briquet's Syndrome, involves a multiplicity of physical complaints that cannot be fully explained or diagnosed and that are not intentionally produced. The complaints start to emerge before the age of thirty and extend over a period of years. The complaints are clinically significant, meaning that they have required medical attention. Often the patient will have a history of medical procedures and treatments that turn out to have been unnecessary. To qualify for this diagnosis, a fairly long list of physical complaints is required: four pain symptoms, two gastrointestinal symptoms, one sexual symptom and one pseudoneurological symptom. A pseudoneurological symptom is a symptom that would ordinarily be connected with a problem in the nervous system, such as vertigo, numbness, paralysis, local weakness, hallucinations, amnesia and so on. Again evaluation does not reveal any underlying physical cause, or if an underlying physical cause is discovered, the reaction of the patient seems to be far in excess of what would be expected from his history and status. The patient is also not feigning sickness for the rewards of the patient role. That is, they are not malingering or suffering from factitious disorder.

5. **Undifferentiated Somatoform Disorder**

If the patient has fewer than the required physical complaints for Somatization disorder, but has had one or more complaints for at least six months, then the diagnosis of Undifferentiated Somatoform Disorder should be considered. Again, the complaints must be clinically significant, that is, they must have entailed medical treatment and, while the complaints are voiced by the patient, there can be found no underlying physical cause. If there is an underlying medical condition, the symptoms and complaints of the patient must be deemed as exceptionally intense and long lasting when related to the diagnosed severity of the condition. The symptoms must also, as in Somatization Disorder, cause impaired functioning in the patient's life. Finally, the disorder should not be better categorized as another somatoform disorder, e.g. Sexual Dysfunction or a Psychotic Disorder, and it must be established that the patient is not intentionally producing the symptoms, that is, it is not Malingering or Factitious Disorder.

6. **Conversion Disorder**

This condition involves disturbances of voluntary sensory or motor functions that cannot be explained by a general medical condition. The disturbances, which can include a long list of sensory problems (numbness, double vision, blindness, deafness, hallucinations and loss of the sensation of pain) and motor problems (loss of balance, weakness, difficulty swallowing, localized paralysis), are brought on by exposure to a psychological stimulus of some sort. For example, the patient may fall over upon seeing a certain person or hearing a certain word or phrase. Sometimes the conversion symptoms may be brought on by the activation of a conflict or unresolved issue. Seizures, fainting or convulsions may also occur as part of this response.

Behavior that is similar to conversion symptoms may be found in certain religious practices. These are not included in this diagnosis. Also these symptoms are not being intentionally created for some sort of gain, nor are they better seen as Pain Disorder or Sexual Dysfunction. These symptoms cause significant impairment in the person's functioning and cannot be explained by any current disease theory. With individuals who are not aware of physiological patterns, the symptoms will frequently go against what is known about the human body and its functioning. For example, the patient may complain of numbness that does not follow the known areas of dermatomes in the human body as, for example, in the instance of "glove anesthesia" where the entire hand is experienced as numb, a phenomenon ruled out by what is known of sensory-motor neural pathways.

7. Pain Disorder

This somatoform disorder has as its main feature a chronic complaint of pain that is serious enough to interfere with the patient's life and warrant medical attention. The pain may or may not be related to an underlying physical condition. Psychological factors are judged to have an important role in the onset and course of the pain. The pain is not intentionally created or feigned. The pain is sufficiently intense to cause problems in work, family and other relationships.

8. Sexual Dysfunction

Clearly, this diagnosis is used when the patient is suffering from a disturbance in their sexual functioning that causes them significant stress or discomfort. There are many types of sexual dysfunction, including dysfunctions having to do with desire, orgasm, pain associated with sexual functioning and problems in sexual functioning related to medical conditions and substance usage.

This is an important area of human functioning. It is complex and affected by multiple factors: age, health, personality, culture and gender, for example. It frequently is difficult for patients and professionals to discuss openly, while it is at the same time an important part of a person's overall sense of well-being. Many physical conditions will be intertwined with sexual functioning. Sometimes as a physical problem is resolved by the clinician, an underlying sexual issue may surface as the patient is now confronted with the possibility of having sex.

9. Hypochondriasis

The distinguishing feature of this condition is the patient having persistent beliefs that she has an illness. The beliefs go on for more than six months and are sufficient enough to disrupt her life, work and relationships in some way. The beliefs are not delusional. That is, she is aware on some level that these ideas may be ill-founded but, despite reassurances from doctors and professionals and the presence of negative findings, she cannot rid herself of the idea that she has an illness--usually a serious one. The concern over health is not about looks primarily (although physical appearance may be involved). If the concern is primarily over appearance (e.g. being too fat or too thin, or balding) then the more appropriate categorization is body dysmorphic disorder.

10. Body Dysmorphic Disorder

The predominant feature of Body Dysmorphic Disorder is a chronic concern with a defect in one's appearance. The patient may feel globally that he is "ugly" or "fat" or he may focus on a specific feature that causes him embarrassment and suffering, such as his buttocks, his watery eyes, his chin or his genitals. He may seek support from others, but the relief provided from this is either non-existent or short-lived. His life becomes constricted as a result of the misperception of his body. This may include limiting social contacts, not going to parties, nor meeting new people, not accepting promotions. Clearly this situation will affect mood and feelings of well-being. The person may have a slight anomaly in his appearance, for example, having slightly thinning hair or a being few pounds overweight, but this small anomaly is magnified into something "repulsive" or "disgusting" or "shameful," to the extent that the patient's life is restricted negatively.

These concerns are above and beyond the usual concerns we find in people of wanting to "look good" and feeling bad when they do not. They manifest chronically and can result in the individual having an aversion to mirrors, or any reflecting surfaces. In addition, these concerns are to be found in persons who otherwise have good contact with reality, and are sometimes marginally aware at times that they "look fine."

11. **Somatoform Disorder Not Otherwise Specified**

This category is reserved for somatoform conditions that do not fit easily into the preceding ten categories. For example, if the somatoform disorder has only been going on for less than six months, it belongs in this category. It also would include instances of *pseudocyesis* (which used to be called hysterical pregnancy) where the patient shows some of the physical signs of pregnancy (enlarged abdomen, reduced menstrual flow and the patient reporting subjective sensations of the fetus moving), but the patient is not pregnant, nor can the condition be explained by other medical means, for example the presence of a tumor or another illness that might cause endocrine changes.

Following is a series of cases to give some practice at thinking about and categorizing these conditions. After, we will consider to what extent some of the psychological theories we have been examining might explain some of these interesting dynamics.

Bill came to the clinic with a sheaf of medical data about his condition. He was attempting, with great difficulty, to get some disability payment to help him get by after an accident in the warehouse where he worked had left him with severe pain in his back that shot down his legs. MRI's showed there was damage to his lumbar vertebrae and his symptoms, although somewhat diffuse and unpredictable, were consistent with the physical findings. He had been prescribed major pain killers but was trying to keep the dosage as low as possible because he did not like the side effects. Bill is wondering whether or not he should add some antidepressants to his regimen because he is having lots of suicidal thoughts recently and is feeling very "low." He is finding that his low spirits are having a negative effect on his family. He is having more fights with his wife and is concerned that his bad moods may be having a negative effect on his ten-year old son, Evan.

The counselor mentioned that it must be very depressing to be undergoing so much stress with the disability claim and there must be sorrow over losing bodily function and not being able to do all the things he used to be able to do. Bill acknowledged that this was true. He had been a very active person before. He even enjoyed social sports like softball with his buddies and rough and tumble games with his son. However, Bill wondered aloud if it was not something deeper. He had always been prone to depression. Perhaps he was even depressed before the accident. "How so?" inquired the counselor. At this Bill opened up that many of his life's dreams had seemed to amount to nothing. All of his projects had failed or had been false starts. He had been identified as a gifted child and had been given many breaks, but somehow they just never bore fruit. He felt he wasn't supposed to end up working in a warehouse. He had actually been part of a doctoral program in Political Science at a prestigious university at one time. When asked how this might have happened, Bill muses that perhaps it had something to do with his father who had abandoned him early on and died soon thereafter. His mother was an alcoholic and an "emotional Vesuvius," blowing up at him for the slightest reason. His three older brothers, seemed to take all their rage out on him. The counselor agreed that this history could well dispose Bill to chronic feelings of depression and low self esteem. It might also, she attempted to tactfully suggest, lead to patterns of unconscious self sabotage. Bill was taken by this idea and wanted to explore further.

*   **Noreen,** a twenty-three-year-old woman, presented several complaints. Among these was a tendency to faint, and a mixing up of words. Both of these caused her considerable concern and embarrassment. She had a complete physical examination and nothing had been found that could physically explain these problems. In addition she had considerable bouts of intense anxiety in social situations that involved dealing with authority figures. These had all worsened recently since she had broken up with her boyfriend of two years and had to move back home.*

*   She had four older brothers and reported that these boys always seemed to get preferential treatment. She had a very intense conflictual relationship with her father whom she tried to avoid at all costs. He is, in her description, a very severe and removed man, anxious about her clothing, as to whether or not it is too revealing, and prone to yelling and physically abusing the mother. He is an isolated man who frequently drinks too much. Noreen reports that her mother is a "flaky" woman who also drinks too much and tries to see the world through rose-colored glasses, sweeping the obvious problems with the father under the rug.*

The brothers have all left home and seem to be living relatively functional, conventional lives. Noreen is struggling to find an identity, it seems. She has tried a few part-time jobs and a few courses at community colleges. The former tend to end in angry conflicts with bosses, while the courses do not seem to be oriented to any clear purpose. Noreen is bright and vivacious some of the time, but when discussing her problems she tears up very easily and becomes very disheartened and confused.

When asked to describe the most recent fainting incident, she tells of how her father tapped on her shoulder when she was washing dishes and curtly told her that it was high time she took out the garbage. Upon examining the fainting episodes, a fairly straightforward pattern emerged. They all involved an interaction with her father in which he invaded her personal space in an unexpected or uninvited way and demanded that she do something. Interestingly, even when discussing this pattern and trying to figure it out in the session, Noreen would flood with feelings and become dizzy, such that the clinician would have to "coach" her through the feelings and sensations with relaxed breathing and focusing on the expression of feelings. Eventually, the intensity of the reactions to discussing these "episodes" abated and it was possible to discuss them relatively calmly. Along with this, Noreen's functioning seemed to improve markedly. Noreen and the clinician then decided to look for similar patterning in her "language problem."

__Audrey__ is a fifty-year-old woman who works in an insurance office as a clerk. She complains of a wide array of intense aches and pains throughout her body, but the worst is in her left leg. She finds it difficult to walk, uses a TENS apparatus and suffers from lack of sleep because of the pain. She lives an isolated life. She reports having no friends and is divorced. Her son lives a few miles away, across town. She reports suffering from what she calls "panic attacks" whenever her boss speaks firmly or critically to her. At these times she will often have to leave work for the rest of the day or sit in the rest room until she calms down.

She is very flat emotionally and does not manifest many feelings, except for physical pain when she has to make certain movements. She has visited many doctors and it appears that they are as frustrated with her as she is with them. Her pain remains a mystery to all concerned since diagnostics show no physical findings.

She is exceedingly sensitive to touch and ready to take emotional offence. It is therefore quite difficult to establish rapport. She seems "prickly," cold and self-protective. Her skin seems cool, as though drained of energy. She looks grim and determined much of the time and very rarely breaks into a smile.

The counselor does her best to try and listen and be helpful but at the end of the session she makes a comment to the effect that the counselor, just like everyone else, only wants to suck money out of her and that maybe it is not worth coming back.

She shows you, at the next session, a piece of art work she did recently at a church workshop. She says it represents how she feels. She is represented as a tiny blob on the wall of a long and winding corridor, deep, deep underground. The corridor, she states, is filled with horrors and there is no way out. When the counselor suggests that it might be nice to take at least an imaginary trip up into the warm sunlight, a look of terror seems to flash across her eyes.

During later sessions, she talks of her mother, with whom she had a very cold and distant relationship. It seems her mother, "Never really wanted her" and hated her, especially after her father, to whom Audrey apparently bears a striking resemblance, left the family for another woman. Her mother seems to prefer Audrey's older sister. Audrey does not get on at all well with her sister either.

Audrey was married, until four years ago, to a man whom she claims was very "aloof and narcissistic" with whom she always felt "alone." Her son seems to be depressed and having trouble establishing an intimate relationship and getting himself established in a career.

Recently, her co-workers gave her a gift certificate to a massage therapist (appropriately named Luz) who seemed to Audrey to have "exactly the right touch." Over the ensuing weeks, Audrey has become very connected to Luz, regarding her as "an angel" and a "lifesaver."

Naomi is a twenty-five-year-old woman who works as a social worker helping the homeless. She has recently moved in with her boyfriend of two years and reports that this relationship is going well for her. She complains of headaches that she thinks come as a result of the intense stress she feels from her work. The organization she works in is very busy these days, since the economy is bad and more people require service. At the same time her pay has been frozen. She also is a very sensitive person and strongly identifies with her clients. While this strong empathic bonding can be a blessing, it also means she tends to take many of her clients problems home with her. She thinks that perhaps if she had some work done on *her back and neck, this would "help her relax" and perhaps relieve the tension headaches. She has seen her general practitioner and he is of the opinion that the headaches are stress related. She likes to converse during the session and she shares that in addition she would like to discuss her relationship with her boyfriend. Generally the relationship is good but often, when he approaches her affectionately in a vigorous manner, she becomes flooded with anxiety and freezes up. He is confused. She then becomes angry and withdrawn and they often have a fight that might go on for a day or two. The relationship improves for a while until the pattern repeats. She says their sexual life is generally satisfactory, although she thinks that maybe she "does not have orgasms, how can you tell?" Eventually, in response to the empathy, interest and concern of the body-worker, Naomi confides that she was sexually abused by an uncle who used to live with her family while she was in grade school. She states she feels silly even bringing it up, because she should know the answer, but perhaps, she wonders aloud, this might have some connection to her relationship with her boyfriend. She responds well to the work done on her neck and back, and this, combined with some stress reduction education helps reduce the frequency and intensity of her headaches.*

Phyllis is a thirty-year-old office manager. She comes to the clinic mostly interested in the pain in her knees and nutritional counseling. After several treatments, the pain abates and she continues to be interested in the nutritional counseling. Slowly, she reveals that she is desperately trying to lose weight because she finds her body "disgusting," even though she thinks she has a pretty face. She acknowledges that she likes to wear very loose fitting clothing so that her "deformity" is not visible. She shares that she would like to have a boyfriend but that this is unlikely to happen until she loses weight. You mention to her that while she is not skinny, she is certainly not obese and that, in your opinion, most men would find her very attractive. She brushes this aside. "While that may be true," she says, " I still cannot help feeling this way about my body." She says she feels imprisoned by her looks. She has a hard time going to parties or other social gatherings because she believes people are staring at her, wondering how she could let herself be seen in public with such a "gross body." She feels quite "low" most of the time, since she has very few friends and sees very little hope of having a significant love relationship in the near future.

Marshall is a twenty-five-year-old graduate student. He dresses very trimly and clearly works out a lot to keep in shape. He has a wide array of complaints—foot pains when he runs and lower back pain that comes and goes for reasons he does not know. As the body-worker talks to him he freely admits that he has strong tendencies to imagine illnesses for himself. He spends hours on the internet investigating the tiniest faults and flaws in his body or even in his thinking. These concerns have been going on for as long as he can recall but seem to have worsened over the past few years. For example, even though he has not had any unsafe sex he was certain last year that he had contracted HIV. It took several tests, repeated several times, to convince himself that this was not the case. He goes on to report several other cases like this, involving his bowels, his urinary tract and his brain. He speaks well and seems quite intelligent. He has a good vocabulary and is very polite in his demeanor. When the body-worker asks him about his family history she finds that his father died when he was six, suddenly, while Marshall was in the room with him. Marshall, as he talks about this seems to tear up, but when you say, "I am sorry, that must have been traumatic and these memories seem to be coming back to you as we speak." He simply states that that is all behind him now and that he has dealt with it. His mother works as a paralegal and, despite having to work very hard, has managed to provide a good life for Marshall and his younger brother, Edward.

Marshall has strong protective feelings towards his mother and evinces annoyance at his brother for stressing the family by being "immature." Marshall would like to go to a good job opportunity in a city some seven hundred miles away, but he is conflicted at leaving his family. He does have a girlfriend of two years and they seem to get on well. He is eager to deal with his foot and back pains, but also would like to address what he calls "over-reactiveness" to his ideas that he might be seriously ill. He knows they are not real, but he cannot get rid of these obsessional thoughts. He also wants to learn to relax, so he is not so easily get upset by small things.

Answers

Bill would probably be categorized as having **Psychological Factors Affecting Medical Condition** insofar as his depression is associated with his physical problems. In addition the depression seems to have been going on a long time and might benefit from some treatment.

Noreen best fits the category of **Conversion Disorder.** Her fainting seems to have no physical cause and is associated with some fairly specific stimuli. It seems to be related to tensions she has in relation to her father.

Audrey can be placed in the category of **Pain Disorder.** She has chronic and dispersed pain throughout her body. It seems that this pain could be related to her troubled relationship to her mother.

Naomi is clearly under a lot of stress and is showing some physical reactions to this. The concern that seems to emerge at the end of the case description, however, is that of **Sexual Dysfunction.** Her sexual enjoyment with her boyfriend is disturbed and she appears to have no orgasms. This is probably related to her sexual abuse.

Phyllis has markedly distorted perceptions of her body. This we would categorize as **Body Dysmorphic Disorder.**

Marshall with his tendency to have imaginary illnesses, would be classed as an example of **Hypochondriasis.**

CHAPTER 14
Difficult People: Personality Disorders in Everyday Practice

Introduction: Personality and Trauma

At the very beginning of this book we examined the theory that traumatic experiences will manifest themselves in bodily symptoms and may resurface in the context of working with the body. Traumatic experiences can also result in what are called in the standard psychological nomenclature, "personality disorders". As van der Kolk explains in "Trauma, the Long Term Effects" (1995), depending on the multiple features of the trauma, a wide array of personality features can result. In one individual, the person may respond by flattening all their feelings. In another, they may develop a profound depression, while in yet another, the response may involve chronic anger and self destructive behavior.

It is therefore quite expectable that the body-worker who is dealing with persons who have been subjected to traumata of various kinds, will, in the course of their work, encounter clients who manifest these pervasive personality adjustments to trauma, that are called personality disorders. We hope that this chapter helps the practitioner identify some of these personalities and understand some of the underlying dynamics. Thus, the body worker might be better able to achieve their goals.

Because physical difficulties happen to people with different personalities and there is a complex interaction between the two. The personality can, at times, precondition the physical problem and the physical problem will at times be affected by the patient's personality. Each person will have a different array of coping styles and these will affect the course of the problem, their way of adapting to it, their relationship to the treatment specialist and the treatment specialist's reaction to them. What follows is a simple beginning sketch-map of this complex terrain.

What is a personality disorder?

One can arrange psychological difficulties on a continuum as we can see in the table below.

Table 1: Spectrum of Psychological Difficulties

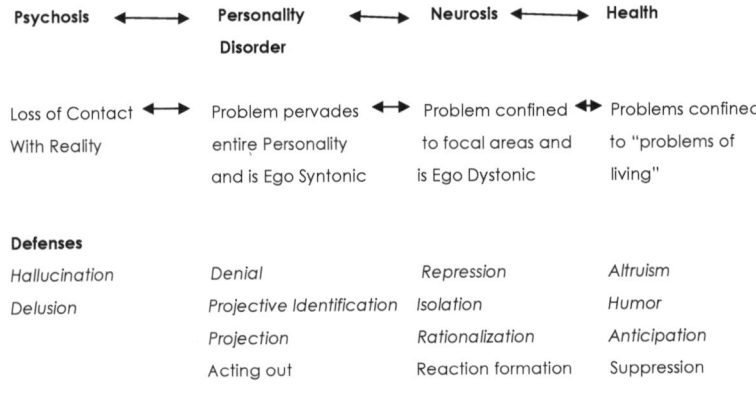

Thus we can see that a personality disorder is not a psychosis. These people are capable of reality testing. They may, at times have unusual ideas, but still hold to the notion of checking the reality of these ideas out with others. We can also see that these difficulties are more serious than a neurosis. Neurotic persons know they have a problem. A personality disorder is when the person has a problem but does not think they do...the problem is in the world.

Personality disorders are usually longstanding forms of adjustment usually go back to childhood. They usually require years of treatment.

At root these can be seen as ways that people are very difficult to live with, by being, among many other things, aggressive, withdrawing, self centered, impulsive, and obsessive.

What can we do?

Psychotherapy has developed some reasonably good ways of working with these problems, but many people with personality disorders do not think they have a problem, so they often do not subject themselves to a long and intensive course of psychotherapy, which is usually what is required.

As healthcare professionals, we will encounter such persons in our practice; perhaps the following will give some insight and some ideas on how to be helpful. At the very least it may ease some of the frustration one often feels in relating to persons with these types of issues.

What are the types?

The Diagnostic and Statistical Manual of Mental Disorders (DSM) has included and dropped in its inventory about a dozen or so different personality disorders over the years. The following list includes most of those that made the list at some time. The list is ever-changing because these are unstable categories. They still can be very useful in helping us chart relationships with others, we find, and in anticipating many of the difficulties encountered in working with people suffering from these painful adjustments. Throughout this section we would like the reader to be aware that these longstanding personality patterns are individuals' attempts to cope, as best they could, with trauma. This helps overcome the pejorative and alienating tone that all-too-often pervades discussion in this domain. Following is a capsule presentation of the key features of each of the types. McWilliams (1994), gives a fine psychodynamically oriented and detailed description.

Narcissistic

Self-centered, entitled
Vulnerable to criticism
Poor at empathy
Grandiosity (often alternating with low self esteem)
Needs to be admired, at the center of attention

Obsessive-Compulsive

Perseverative, has trouble ending things
Gets stuck on details
One track mind
Cannot get thoughts out of head (Hypochondriasis)

Dependent

Difficulty being on their own
Easily influenced by others
Compromises values to be with others

Borderline

Easily provoked by frustration, let downs
Chronic anger.
Very sensitive to abandonment and imposition of boundaries
Poor object constancy
Can switch quickly from idealizing to denigrating others

Paranoid

Suspicious, plotting
Isolated
Often intellectual
Often selects jobs where hypervigilance and suspicion are needed.

Schizoidal

Emotionally flat
Prefers things to people
Enjoys being alone
Poor empathy

Schizotypal

Bizarre ideas and language
Not delusional, but strange world views.

Antisocial

Lack of concern for others, rules and laws
Empathy only in pursuit of self interest

Histrionic

Drama king/queen
Superficial relationships to self and others
Sexually seductive/love triangles

Avoidant

Longs to be with others but has social anxiety
Loneliness, low self esteem

Passive Aggressive/Self Defeating

Self sabotage
Wet blanket
Help rejecting complainer

How will they respond to treatment?

Each type will have a different reaction to physical disability and to being in treatment. Each will have different ways of coping with the stress. Many of these ways will make treatment more difficult than usual. Following is a listing of some typical difficulties to be expected.

Narcissistic

Will feel low self esteem
Will expect special treatment
Will feel insulted by the process

Obsessive/compulsive

May tend towards hypochondriasis
Will have trouble seeing the forest for the trees...gets lost in details
Trouble completing things
Pickiness

Dependent

Will have trouble following through on their own
Will have problems if cure means more independence
Will tend to go along with whatever others say
Have trouble making up his own mind

Borderline
Will tend to get into conflicts, especially if they feel abandoned
Oftentimes will have trouble with independent functioning
Can make unrealistic demands on time and get angry when these are not met.

Paranoid
Will tend to be suspicious and non-trusting
Could be litigious
May become an "expert in the field" and second guess your judgment
May play you off against others

Schizoidal
Might be hard to connect with emotionally
Might be hard to read, to know how they are feeling
Slow to warm up

Schizotypal
Some ideas and attitudes might seem far out and off-putting
Reactions to treatment might seem bizarre at times
Use of language might be idiosyncratic and need explaining, e.g. new words that have private meaning

Antisocial
Maybe ethical dilemmas over rules they break
Anxiety at being with someone who breaks rules
Possible involvement of judicial system

Avoidant
Sometimes treatment may require social interaction
Hard to get them to open up and relax with you
Sometimes getting better proves problematic because they can be expected to be more social

Histrionic
Intense reactions to small things can be hard to read. Are they really in that much pain?

Intense emotionality may interfere with more down to earth aspects of treatment

Personal life might be tumultuous and interfere with treatment

Passive Aggressive

Complaining and rejection of help can be frustrating

Complaining and sabotaging of treatment can stir up resentment

Lack of gratitude or acknowledgement of treatment can be frustrating

Examples

The following capsules are aimed at giving you a feel for each of the types. This is just a beginning to understanding. Each of these characters will have a unique history that explains their genesis. we highly recommend Nancy McWilliam's text (1994) on the psychodynamics of personality disorders for one approach to understanding these often difficult individuals.

> A. *Doris is 28 years old, currently unemployed and suffers from pain in her lower back. She reports a history of substance abuse and a series of conflicts with her bosses. She also reports having difficulties with her current boyfriend. The first treatment went very well and she thought you were an angel from heaven. Something you said during the second session set her off, however, and she is very angry at you now, having called you two times for an explanation before she returns to the clinic. You are not sure what it was you said.*

> B. *Harold is a 42-year-old male. Never married, he seems to complain and whine about everything. He has seen a series of people and they were all no good for him, they didn't understand him and asked too much of him. He seems to find everything too difficult, even quailing at the simplest of exercise regimens. You are starting to feel frustrated yourself. If only he would meet you half way. You feel drained at the end of the session.*

C. *Hermione is a fifty-year-old woman. She dresses much more nicely than necessary to visit the clinic and seems to look down on the other patients. She asks if there is a way she could be moved to the front of the line, since she has some very important appointments. She speaks frequently of the important people she has met and the interesting places she has been. She seems to deny that she has some serious physical problems, as if this would be something that is beneath her.*

D. *Archibald, a 58-year-old man, is very pleasant and smiles at all around him. He suffered an injury some five years ago and explains it as a message from the angels amongst us. He writes poetry that he recites at a local coffee bar every month and wears amulets of his own design. Every now and then he will look you in the eyes so he can "read your inner being." He has a job, cleaning in a local store, and is not taking any psychotropic medication.*

E. *Beth is a 45-year-old woman who was hit in the back by a laundry cart in the laundromat parking lot. She is small in stature and pale. She responds to questions with brief factual answers and not much emotion at all. In fact when she reported that she would have to miss a week of treatment because her mother was very ill, and you said, "That must be hard for you." She simply responded with, "I suppose." It is hard to read her feelings and develop a relationship with her. She works as a computer technician. When you ask her about work, she responds mostly in terms of the technical problems she faces, not the people she works with.*

F. *Brett is a 35-year-old electronics technician. He arrives with a sheaf of notes on his condition and takes notes while you are talking to him. He wipes the seat before he sits on it and insists you spray the head-rest twice to kill the germs* and fungus. He admits to a tendency to imagine illnesses, but says no matter how hard he tries, he cannot get the thoughts out of his head. When you give him some exercise instructions at the end of the session, it takes a long time for him to understand, simply because he gets lost in the details and can't seem to grasp the general idea.

G. Bertrand is 45-years-old and unemployed. He is lively and states that one of the reasons he has problems is that he is a bit of a thrill-seeker and gets bored easily. He was dishonorably discharged from the military and has had a few stints in jail. On his second visit he offers to sell you a watch that he reports, with a wink, he found. He owes you some money for sessions, sessions that he says he needs for a lawsuit he is pursuing. So far, there appear to be no discernible physical problems with him.

H. Elise is warm and expressive. She calls the entire staff "darling" and flirts with the male nurse and seems hurt when he is unresponsive and simply professional. She seems to have a tumultuous personal life and this leads to her changing appointments frequently. Physical treatments are difficult because she has such strong reactions sometimes to things that seem small. The slightest tweak will give her "terrors" or "keep her up all night." She likes to be the center of attention, often wearing provocative clothing, and seems to pout when she feels ignored. She is not cold or mean, but seems not to remember important things about others. She forgets, for example, that she has asked you three times already how many children you have.

I. Egbert is quiet, like "Casper Milquetoast" jokes one of the assistants. He follows instructions and is timely and polite, but when you assign some leg exercises for him he seems to balk, almost as if he might have trouble standing on his own two feet. One day he says something odd: when you ask him

"How do you feel?" He replies' "How should I feel?" as if to ask permission for a feeling.

J. *Bill is a 45-year-old lawyer. His body is extremely tense and his blood pressure very high. When you ask him how things are going at work, he says, "Why do you need to know that?" with suspicion. He finally does talk about work and shares that he thinks most people are trying to "bring him down," "After all," he continues, "it is a dog eat dog world." He checks your credentials closely and goes over the bill with you. He also spends a good deal of time asking you questions about your background, training, lawsuits you have had and with whom you share the treatment information. He tells you he wants to be notified of any changes in treatment that he should know about beforehand. You agree to do this.*

K. *Biff is brought to the clinic by his mother. She is sure he has a physical problem of some sort. Why else would a young man of 19 never leave his room except to go to the bathroom? Biff is very quiet. He reads a lot of sci-fi and is into video games. His lack of physical exercise has lead to obesity and chronic back and muscle problems. When you suggest getting out and exercising he becomes very uncomfortable. After a while he opens up a bit and shares that he is very lonely and shy. He used to have a friend in grade school, but he moved to Florida and since then it has been torture for him to go out in public. He would like to go to college, maybe the gym, but he is very anxious in these social situations.*

Answers:

Recalling again, the many difficulties involved in categorizing people, here are the answers that we think provide the best fit. Also please recall that diagnosis is an ongoing process. These assessments will change as we learn more about the person.

A. *Doris seems to fit the borderline category. She*

is prone to anger, self medicates and switches quickly from idealization to denigration.

B. Harold seems to fit the category of passive aggressive personality. He seems invested in undermining the process of treatment. He is perhaps angry, but has difficulty in expressing it directly and effectively.

C. Hermione seems to be narcissistic. She expects special treatment, seems grandiose and is self centered.

D. Archibald seems to be schizotypal. He has unusual ideas and it is difficult to get into everyday contact with him. However, he is in touch with everyday reality.

E. Beth could be categorized as schizoidal. She is emotionally flat and removed. She seems to prefer things to people.

F. Brett seems to be obsessive-compulsive. He gets lost in the details and suffers from fixed ideas and hypochodriasis.

G. Bertrand, with his tendency to break the law and thrill seeking seems to fit the bill for an antisocial personality.

H. Elise's effusiveness and seductiveness seem to place her in the category of histrionic personality. She also has intense reactions to small stimuli and does not seem to relate to others in a deep manner.

I. Egbert seems quite "other directed" and susceptible to peer pressure. This would place him in the category of dependent personality for the time being.

J. Bill's suspiciousness and tendency to file lawsuits inform us that he may be somewhat paranoid.

K. Biff seems lonely. He wants friends and misses them, but he has social anxiety. This would place him in the avoidant category.

CHAPTER 15

The Theory of Positive Disintegration and Working with the Body

This chapter intends to show how the body may be related to the processes of emotional development described in the theory of positive disintegration developed by Dabrowski (1970,1977). The fundamental idea is that the process of maturation involves an important, but potentially disruptive, disintegration of psychological structures, structures that must dissolve and be reorganized if a new and more complex arrangement is to grow. We argue that body-work, insofar as it might loosen repressions, evoke memories and open the mind can be a potentiator of such a positive disintegration. The body-worker may thus find herself midwife to such processes. Often these processes are pathologized—people see the increased intensity of feeling or the confusion as something that is wrong with them and try to get rid of it. This is unfortunate for such feelings can pave the way to richer more complex living. This topic is addressed in some more detail in the book, "The Experience of Emptiness." It thus behooves the body-worker to be aware of these developmental processes so that they may flourish. First we will describe the theory of positive disintegration.

The Theory of Positive Disintegration
The Levels of Development

Level I - Primary Integration:

At this level the person is organized around the meeting of basic survival needs. The person at this stage feels relatively well integrated and has as his primary purpose the meeting of "instinctual needs," e.g. hunger, sex, safety, shelter, comfort. It seems as though the person is dealing primarily with what Maslow (1968) termed "basic needs" and not "meta-needs," or higher level needs. The individual at this level of development is unaware of meta-needs, or if he is aware of them, assimilates them to his or her primary orientation of meeting basic needs. This would occur in much the same fashion that Kohlberg (1981) has demonstrated that people of lower levels of moral development interpret and assimilate the acts of higher moral development entirely in the terms of lower moral development. That is, for example, they may interpret altruistic acts as being acts of meeting basic needs. Level I is the level of the confident, unconflicted, self-serving individual. They are untroubled by a complex or a deep concern for others.

Level II - Unilevel Disintegration:

At this level the relatively smooth functioning of Level I breaks up, disintegrates and leaves the person with a predominantly wavering attitude. The previously well-bound and integrated structure now becomes loose, resulting in the individual feeling attacks of directionlessness and chaos. There is a difficulty in making decisions; forces within the person push against one another so that the person vacillates. In the absence of an internal hierarchical organization (the disintegration is unilevel) the forces do not resolve into smooth and deliberate action. The person at this stage is very subject to polarities of emotion. Sometimes the disintegration can be extreme and result in substance abuse or even psychosis. In other instances, the person can "pull themselves together" and manage to function in a seemingly integrated way. Under pressure, however, the disintegration returns. Frequently people at this stage long for a return to the "good old days" of Primary Integration, when things seemed, by comparison, simple. The words of Yeats' poem (1989) seem to capture Unilevel Disintegration quite aptly:

"Things fall apart, the center cannot hold,
Mere anarchy is loosed upon the world."

The hallmarks of this level are other-directedness, ambivalence, mixed feelings, ambitendency, confused and conflictual activity, and the sense of having multiple selves. The individual is unsure as to what is really important, as to what should take precedence.

Level III - Spontaneous Multilevel Disintegration:

At this level of development, things are still fallen apart, but there is a growing hierarchization within the person. Instead of equipotent forces acting upon each other, resulting in a wavering, vacillating directionlessness, there is a developing sense of a hierarchy of values, with certain values and forces emerging as prepotent. The person begins to feel "inferiority towards himself," that is, he starts to experience the difference between what he is and what he ought to be. This develops out of the newly-emerging hierarchy of aims and values. Among some of the other "dynamisms" (or experiences that can facilitate and encourage further development) are: positive maladjustment, feelings of guilt, feelings of shame, astonishment with oneself, hierarchization, subject-object in oneself, inner psychic transformation and self-awareness, self-control, autopsychotherapy and education-of-oneself.

Level IV - Organized Multilevel Disintegration:

In this stage the person has developed an organized and consistent hierarchy within him or herself. In the words of Ogburn (1976):

"He has transcended the problem of becoming
And tackles the problems of being." (Ogburn, 1976)

The basic needs are generally well taken care of at this stage or have receded into the background; the individual is concerned largely with the meta-needs that Maslow speaks of. (Maslow, 1968, p. 210) In fact, Piechowski argues that there is a strong correspondence between the Self Actualizing person of Maslow's thinking and the person who has achieved Level IV. Thus, some of the active dynamisms are: self-awareness, knowledge of one's uniqueness, developmental needs, existential responsibility, self-control, regulating one's own development, education-of-oneself, self-induced programs of systematic development. The primary task of the individual at this stage of development is to solidify the structure that emerges from the previous disintegrated stage.

The locus of control (that is, whether they feel they are directed from within themselves or without) for the individual at Level IV is very firmly an internal one--he or she can act independently of the external environment if he so chooses.

Level V – Secondary Integration:

Only a few rare individuals reach this level of development. At this stage, the "ought" has become unified with "what is." The personality ideal has been achieved. The planful self-development of Level IV has been successfully completed. Individuals at this level seem to experience self, other, time, being and the world in radically different ways. Thus, persons at the other levels often have difficulty understanding them.

Overexcitabilities

Development through the stages is related, in large part, to the level and profile of excitabilities in the person. Dabrowski posits five types of overexcitabilities: Emotional, Psychomotor, Sensual, Intellectual and Imaginational. An overexcitability is a predisposition in the individual, largely inherited, to respond to certain types of stimuli in an above average manner. For example, a person with sensual overexcitability will be more responsive than average to cutaneous stimulation. He or she will also tend, if this tends to be his or her dominant type of overexcitability, to transform other types of experience, (e.g., emotional, intellectual, imaginational) into sensual types of experience. For example, the emotion of affection will be readily transformed into stroking for a person with sensual overexcitability.

Perhaps another term for overexcitability would be sensitivity, perhaps analogous to photographic paper which can be varied in its sensitivity to various types of light input. The pronounced overexcitability would correspond to a finely grained, highly sensitized paper--the impression of reality gained when there is an overexcitability that is correspondingly sharp, intense and vivid.

Following is a brief overview of the manifestations of the various forms of overexcitabilities (OEs):

Sensual: This manifests through a heightened sensitivity to sensual experience—skin stimulation, sexual excitability, the desire for stroking, physical comfort, tastes, sights, colors, etc.

Psychomotor: This manifests itself in a tendency for vigorous movement, violent games and sports, rapid talk and a pressure to be moving. Emotional excitement is converted into movement that is highly charged with energy. Dancers and athletes might have a high degree of this OE.

Imaginational: This is shown in sensitivity to the imagined possibilities of things. There is a rich association of images and metaphors flow freely. People with high levels of this OE might easily confuse reality and imagination.

Intellectual: In this the individual displays a voracious curiosity and desire to learn and understand. There is a persistence in asking probing questions and a reverence for logic. There is a love of theory and an intense enjoyment of thinking.

Emotional: This is the most important overexcitability in that if this is absent or weak, it is unlikely that development will proceed. Emotional overexcitability is manifested in the person's ability to form strong emotional attachments to others, and living things and places. Also present with emotional overexcitability are: concern about death, strong affective memory, concern for others, empathy, exclusive relationships and feelings of loneliness. People with high levels of this OE often say they are "too emotional."

The level of development the individual reaches is dependent upon three factors. The **first factor** is the person's hereditary endowment, namely, the configuration of his overexcitabilities and other genetic inheritances. The **second factor** is the environment in which the individual lives and the extent to which it supports or impedes that individual's development, for example, family, school, community. The **third factor** consists of the individual's response to his or her situation—the decisions he or she makes in response to the life situation he finds himself in and the genetic heritage that he possesses.

The **third factor** is only found significantly at Level III or above, that is, persons at levels I and II are molded entirely by genetic, constitutional and environmental factors. Only at Level III does the individual start to take hold of their situation (in an almost "existential" way) and make a conscious, self-determined choice as to how they will act.

Equipped with this brief overview of TPD (the theory of positive disintegration) let us now examine how some of these ideas might apply to body work.

Case Example: Henry, falling to pieces to come together again.

Henry, a 42-year-old psychology professor came to a massage therapist because he was given a gift certificate by a friend. He went thinking it would go along nicely with his psychotherapy since he had been feeling a sort of emptiness in his life. He was successful and healthy, made good money and was happily married. However, something was missing. As the massage proceeded he found himself shivering and feeling intense coldness. The room was, in fact, very warm so the sensation was a mystery. The therapist simply stated that this was not that uncommon and he should perhaps stay with the feelings. Eventually the shivering and cold gave way to a soothing, deep warmth and he lapsed into a deep relaxation. This was a mystery to him. He decided to continue with the massage. Each time the shivering returned but with shorter and shorter durations. Simultaneously, he was working on the strange emptiness he felt in his life. One weekend he found himself crying and crying for an hour or two, on his own and with no obvious reason. He believed it was as if something deep had been loosened in him but he did not know what, some sadness that he had been split off from for a long time. He felt extremely confused and disorganized. This was not like him. He was usually the most rational of people. A flash of free association gave him a clue. He suddenly, for no apparent reason recalled a cartoon he had seen as a child of the story of the "Snow Queen," where a small boy meets the snow queen. She puts a shard of ice in his heart and it prevents him from having any feelings ever again. He abandons his childhood friend and wanders off to the Queen's ice palace in the frozen north. Only love finally melts the shard of ice in his heart and he rejoins his loved ones. Henry wondered who or what had frozen his heart. The only thing that came to his mind was that he had lost his beloved grandmother to a sudden illness when he was very young. He could not remember this, but perhaps his body did. Perhaps he had frozen his heart. Perhaps the massage and the psychotherapy had melted the ice shard. Whether or not this was true, Henry's life certainly changed. Friends started not to know him. He welled up with feelings at music, movies, meetings. He had emotional outbursts. He fell in love. He went to pieces; not in a "bad" way, but in a way that puzzled both him and his friends. He knew he had many years of work ahead of him to reconstruct his new self.

This case serves to illustrate just one way in which some otherwise mysterious process can be explained using the template of the theory of positive disintegration. The process of growth is not always in a smooth line,. Just as we might have to endure a period of disorganization when we rehab a house, so we might have to go through a period of positive disintegration as we grow to new levels of psychological complexity.

The theory of positive disintegration (TPD) would also seem to imply that an individual would have a different relationship to body-work depending on their level and on their profile of overexcitabilities. For example an individual at level one might find it very difficult to let go and allow him or herself a range of emotional responses to body-work. She might also be threatened by the loss of control or of feelings of vulnerability that are sometimes associated with body-work. We are of the opinion that many individuals who might appear to be level one only appear that way because rigidification is a common response to trauma. Again, body-work, which seeks flexibility and motility can loosen such traumatic adaptations, and, again, the individual at level one will be especially unnerved by this.

Individuals at level two will perhaps manifest in body-work many of the characteristics of that level. They may display ambivalence and ambitendency towards the work, on the one hand seeking self renewal and exploration and then, just as quickly reversing direction. To the unprepared body-worker, this may seem surprising. In addition, individuals at level two are themselves concerned at the multiplicity of their "many selves." Persons at level two are also "other directed" and this may influence the work insofar as they may be more concerned with how they come across to others—how they look, and how others may evaluate them. They may, in consequence, have difficulties arriving at their own independent assessments of who they are, what they feel and what they want.

At level three, we may witness in the individual a connection of the body to more inchoate strivings. Individuals at this level may report mystical experiences in the course of body-work. However, they will be unable, as yet, to integrate them fully into a meaningful system. They may then feel very guilty or inferior as a result of this discrepancy between the "lower" everyday parts of themselves and these more "exalted" experiences that they are prone to.

The individual at level four is in a much more integrated frame of mind. They arrive at an integrated view of self, body and mind that results in a celebration and acceptance of the infinite complexity of the body. They approach body-work with an openness to new experiences of self and other and seem to take the disruption of new learnings in their stride.

Similarly, clients with different overexcitabilities (OE's) will respond tpo body-work in very different ways. Those with intellectual OE will seek the logic of their reactions and will perhaps look for the science behind the work. Those with sensual OE will respond strongly to the touch, contact and rubbing. Those with psychomotor OE will perhaps prefer more vigorous types of body-work and may find it hard to lie still for prolonged periods of time. Those with imaginational OE may respond to body-work with images or visions or sounds or novel ideas running through their heads. Finally, those with emotional OE will respond with feelings, memories of relationships and will be more likely to form an emotional attachment to the body-worker.

We hope that this précis of TPD alerts the reader to yet more complexity in the responses of clients to body-work.

Section V
Creating a Growth-Facilitating Environment

Clearly, one of the major ideas in this book is that there is a significant psychological factor involved in all body-work and that the professional body-worker, if they are to be fully effective, should be aware of this and ready to respond appropriately to such phenomena in their clients. This section provides some beginning ideas and guidelines on what body-workers might do in responding to their clients and in establishing a growth promoting environment in the institutions in which they function.

CHAPTER 16:

Growth-Promoting Responses: Carl Rogers Theory

Professionals who have not been trained in basic counseling skills are often at a loss when their clients show emotions or share their problems. Throughout this book we have argued that such sharing is to be expected when working with the body. We will now examine one of the most basic and useful of theories of counseling—a theory that has been widely tested and validated and a theory that is reasonably easily mastered—the client centered theory of Carl Rogers. Here, we will only provide the basic scaffolding of the theory. We strongly suggest interested readers to explore further. Rogers' books are widely available and readable (1961).

Diagram 14 gives a visual of our understanding of the basic concepts in Rogers' theory. At the center of the process is the ***organism***. This is everything you are—your ideas, feelings, your body, your hopes, dreams—the "real" of the organism itself. The organism is a process, continually unfolding and we are continually learning new aspects of the organism if we are growing, if we are fully functioning.

Diagram 14: Carl Rogers' Personality Theory

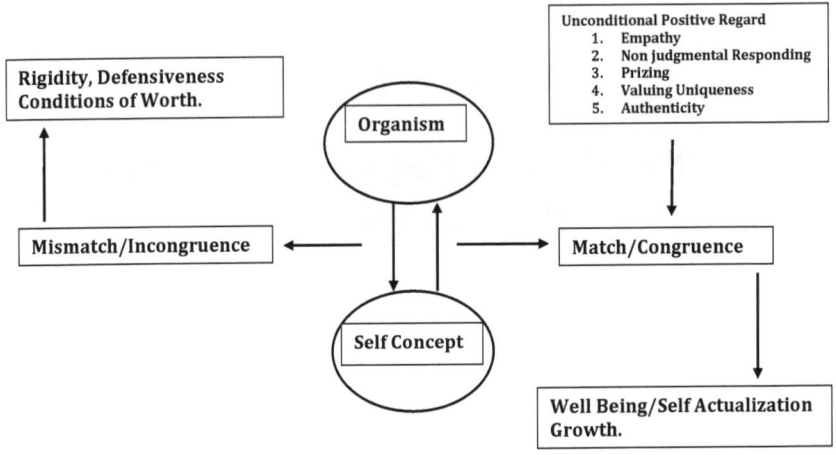

Unconditional Positive Regard
1. Empathy
2. Non judgmental Responding
3. Prizing
4. Valuing Uniqueness
5. Authenticity

Rigidity, Defensiveness
Conditions of Worth.

Organism

Mismatch/Incongruence

Match/Congruence

Self Concept

Well Being/Self Actualization
Growth.

We form an image of our organism and this is called the **self concept.** This is the set of ideas, beliefs and cognitions we form about the nature of our organism. It would involve ideas like, "I never cry," or, "I sometimes lose my temper," or, "I never give in." Clearly some of these ideas about the organism will match, that is, they are truthful statements about the organism, and sometimes they will not match. When there is a match-up between the self concept and the organism, it is called **congruence**, when there is a mismatch, it is called **incongruence.** Incongruence is uncomfortable. It results in tension, rigidity, anxiety and defensiveness. We tend to feel out of touch with ourselves, like we are putting on a mask. It is harder to let go and be free and spontaneous. We are probably more careful than we need to be in interpersonal situations. In all likelihood, this tension and "out-of-touchness" will show up in the body, for the body is part and parcel of the organism. This incongruence results in a stasis. It becomes difficult to grow and realize our full potential, because we are out of touch with our true selves, our organism. Incongruence also results in **conditions of worth**, in other words, we have fluctuations in self esteem. When we convince ourselves that our self concept and organism are meshing we feel good about ourselves. When we become aware that the mask is slipping and we become aware that our preferred self concept is not matching our organism (for example, when the organism cries and our self concept contains the scripting that we never cry) we tend to feel lowered self esteem.

Under the fortunate circumstances of **congruence** the situation is different. Self esteem does not fluctuate; in fact, it probably becomes an irrelevant concept because the self concept simply reflects the here-and-now reality of the organism without judgments being cast. The individual feels a relaxed self acceptance and is primed for growth because they are in touch with the reality of their fully functioning organism. In all likelihood, this is reflected in bodily states.

Clearly, congruence is the more desirable state so the question arises, "How does one create an environment where congruence is more likely to occur?" The answer is that one must provide **unconditional positive regard.** This is comprised of five elements. Together these elements provide an environment where the individual finds it easier to make accurate links between their self concept and their organism. The five elements that make up unconditional positive regard are: empathy, non judgmental responding, prizing, valuing uniqueness and authenticity. Volumes have been written on these. Following is a brief summary.

Empathy involves accurately reflecting back to the person what they seem to be sensing, thinking and, importantly, feeling. This is not sympathy, which involves an element of pity. It is an straightforward attempt to show the other that you have accurately registered their unique experience at that moment. It sounds simple, but it requires discipline. For example, it demands that one listen, not jump to conclusions, offer premature advice or ask unnecessary questions, just listen.

Non judgmental Responding means to respond in such a way that the person feels psychologically safe, safe from criticism or put downs. This often requires care in selecting one's words. One might have to develop a knack for using words that are value neutral, for example, if a person says, "I am such a mean person!" it could be responded to with, "You feel under pressure, and you feel you have to take care of yourself." This response would perhaps be seen as empathic and non-judgmental. The individual will feel safer to open up, to make more accurate connections between their self concept and their organism.

Prizing is a deceptively simple concept. It simply means paying close attention to the other, making them, in that moment, the center of your world so they feel valued and worthy. This encourages self exploration for reinforces the idea that they are a valuable individual, worthy of curiosity, of exploration. Having a hurried schedule, looking at one's watch, being distracted, not making eye contact, coming off through one's body language as distant and uninvolved all undermine this feeling of being prized.

Valuing uniqueness is, we believe a rather radical assumption. Its radicality emerges as one explores it further. The organism is, of course, unique. One occupies a unique place in space and time. One's experience is unique, resistant to categorization. As such it remains mysterious to oneself and others. Thus when we attempt to categorize others or depersonalize them, or place them in a group, we do damage to the congruence that could exist between the self concept and the organism. In addition, people will damage their own sense of uniqueness. It is not at all uncommon for people to enter one of our clinics having already labeled themselves as "bipolar" or "a disability case". These labels are extremely risky insofar as they run roughshod over the uniqueness of each individual's response to these situations. Clinicians should thus be very careful not to "rubricize" not to too easily place clients into categories. This can be overcome to some extent by showing curiosity about the client's unique response to his situation, whatever it might be.

Authenticity means being real about your own organismic responding. While, as professionals, we are paid not to inflict our worries and concerns on others who come to us for help, it is important that we offer that help in an authentic fashion. If we put up a false front, for example, pretending to be "fine" when we are "stressed out and crabby", how can we expect a client to get in touch with the reality of their body, of their organism, of their self? Authenticity means, in addition, being available to one's clients. Again, this is not to be done in such a manner as to flood the client, but if, for example a client should ask, "How was your Thanksgiving?" a response with some authentic sharing, above and beyond the cliché of "Just fine." Might help the client make further contact with their own process.

When these elements are put together, they form a matrix in which the client can form more accurate representations of themselves and in which growth can take place. Given that the organism is so fundamentally a bodily phenomenon, these ideas should be of great use to body-workers.

CHAPTER 17:

Social Systems Theory: Creating a Health-Promoting Institutional Environment for Body-work

Just as it is important for the body-worker to provide a health-promoting relationship on an individual, interpersonal level, it also vital that the institutional context in which the body-work takes place does the same. In this section, we will briefly describe some key ideas that might help in the development and maintenance of a health-promoting organization.

There is a vast literature on organizational health and what we present here is, of course drawn from some of these writings. We present these ideas in the form of a checklist so that the practitioner may run through them and evaluate the health of their institution.

A key variable affecting organizational health that is noted by Chris Argyris (1995) is **discussability.** This idea has to do with the extent to which the very organization itself is discussable. If members feel relatively free to talk about the processes they experience in the organization and how it feels to work there it is generally a good sign, especially if they believe that what they say will be listened to. It betokens openness to self examination in the institution and often implies a willingness to change.

What might be useful things for people in the institution to discuss? We have found that the following acronym can be helpful, "FABART Rules". The acronym stands for:

Fantasies
Affect
Boundaries
Authority
Roles
Tasks
Rules

These ideas have been covered in some detail by Hazell (2005, 2006) but we will cover them briefly here.

Fantasies can be conscious or unconscious. In some clinics we have seen workers who seemed to be engaged in a competition as to who was the favorite of the person in charge, as if he possessed some magical qualities. In others we have seen fantasies expressed about the clientele, their behavior and motivations. Often, these fantasies are not shared or checked out in reality. Often they can interfere with effective work.

Affect has to do with emotions, moods and feelings. We have seen institutions where people seemed to be working under a sort of malaise. In others the mood was upbeat and hopeful. Sometimes these affects can facilitate the work, at others they can clearly get in the way. If they are open to examination they can be studied and, if necessary, changed so as to be more functional.

Boundaries are very crucial in the functioning of organizations. They exist in every phase of work. What are the boundaries like between the workers, professionals and clients? Are they permeable, impermeable, fuzzy, clear, cold, warm, secure or insecure? When we examine the boundaries are they likely to facilitate the task or undermine it? Why are the boundaries kept the way they are? Sometimes they are kept the way they are because of fantasies (conscious or unconscious). We can see how each of the items on this checklist relates to every other item.

Authority has to do with the nature and mobilization of power in the institution. Who has authority? How is it maintained? Should those who have authority in fact have it? Are there those in the organization who have high levels of responsibility but low levels of authority? These people are often called "coordinators" and they are usually stressed out. Is the leadership matched to the task and the individuals being led? Is there appropriate use of participation, delegation, persuasion and so on?

Roles can be formal or informal. Formally, one would ask if all the roles needed are in place. In some clinics we have studied, for example, there was a notable lack of an office manager, a specialist in administration. Thus these tasks fell through the cracks with ensuing chaos, demoralization and confusion. In addition, one may ask whether or not the role is being filled by the right person. Someone may have the role of "manager" but not be personally suited for such a detail-oriented, organizational type of role.

Roles can also be informal. It is usually useful to examine these critically. For example, one individual may play the role of "mother hen" to calm and placate the nerves of people, while another may play the role of the group's "conscience" as if they are some sort of moral arbiter. It may be that the organization needs to have these functions performed, but are they being performed in a way that is most effective for the institutions goals? Many roles occur as a result of **scapegoating**. This process is discussed in Hazell(2005). It is also addressed in this text in the chapter on group and family dynamics. In this process, it is as if the organization unconsciously asks one of its members (or a subset of its members) to hold and express in some form or another, emotions that the group as a whole finds it hard to deal with. This individual then becomes problematic in some way and the group deals with them ambivalently. This process is much more likely to occur in organizations that are under stress, such as that which occurs when there is radical change, especially if the very existence of the organization is threatened. This process is beautifully described by Wells (1985).

In addition, body-workers often work in an atmosphere that is charged with affect. People are in pain, frightened or depressed at the changes and difficulties they are having with their bodies. Menzies Lyth (1960) describes how this very anxiety can result in some **social defense mechanisms** that, while they may reduce the psychological pain experienced consciously (at least for a while) will perhaps compromise the effectiveness of the organization. For example, one of these defense mechanisms is **depersonalization.** In this, we see the workers in a health care institution treating others and even themselves as non-persons, perhaps referring to them as a number, or by the room they occupy, or as a condition. Clearly if one lacks this emotional contact with one's clients one feels a great deal less anxiety. On the other hand much of the effectiveness of the the relationship, becomes severely compromised. Another social defense mechanism is **diffusion of responsibility**. Unfortunately, we have witnessed this also all too frequently in clinics that house body-workers. Again, it is as if the anxiety of working with people who are sick or in pain is so great that the group decides that this is best dealt with if the responsibility for the work is distributed in a vague way over a number of people. Thus, if anything should go wrong, no one individual bears the terrible brunt of responsibility. The buck stops nowhere. Again, while this may be functional to some extent insofar as it enables people to do tasks they might otherwise find too frightening, if carried too far it can seriously undermine performance and lead to deterioration in client relationships, when no-one "steps up to the plate."

Rules obviously have to do with the regulation of behavior of the institution. Are these open for discussion and evaluation? Who sets them? Why are they there? How do they relate to the tasks of the institution? How are they enforced? Who enforces them? What are some of the fantasies about the rules? On and on these questions can go, and this leads us back to the dimension of discussability. If these dimensions can be discussed from time to time in the institution, it bodes well for its health and its functioning. If not, the organization is rolling the dice and hoping for good luck, which is probably not a strategy to be consciously at least, preferred, especially when the stakes are so high.

Finally, we believe that an organization that is devoted in some structural form to the ongoing growth and development of its members is likely to be a more healthy one. Thus we would expect to see in a healthy organization, programs, formal and informal aimed at facilitating the learning, growth, personal and professional development of all the members of that organization. Organizations manifest **parallel process.** If an organization or an individual wishes to foster growth, then the organization and the individual must be themselves growing. If the organization and the individuals comprising it are stagnant, then it cannot expect to foster growth and development amongst its clientele.

References and Further Reading

Argyris, C. and Schon, D. 1995, *Organizational Learning II: Theory, Method and Practice.* FT Press.

Benson, H. 2000, *The Relaxation Response,* Harper Paperbacks.

Bion, W. 1959, "Attacks on Linking," *Second Thoughts,* London, Heinemann (1967)

_____, 1961, *Experiences in Groups,* London, Tavistock.

Birdwhistell, R, 1970, *Kinesics and Context,* University of Pennsylvania Press.

Breuer, J. and Freud, S. (2000/ 1885) *Studies on Hysteria,* Basic Books (Reissue Edition)

Cherniss, Cary. 1980, *Professional Burnout in Human Service Organizations.* Prager.

Clynes, M. 1989, *Sentics, the Touch of the Emotions,* Avery Publishing Group.

Colman, A.D. and Bexton, W.H. (eds) 1975, *Group Relations Reader,* Washington, DC, A.K. Rice Institute.

Colman, A.D. and Geller, W.H. (eds) 1985), *Group Relations Reader 2,* Washington, DC, A.K. Rice Institute.

Csiksentmihalyi, M, 2008, *Flow: The Psychology of Optimal Experience,* Harper Perrenial Modern Classics.

Dabrowski, K., Kawczak, A., Piechowski, M., (1970),*Mental Growth through Positive Disintegration*, Gryf, London.

Dabrowski, K. and Piechowski, M.M., 1977 *Theory of Emotional Development,* Dabor, Oceanside, New York.

Daruna, J. 2004, *Introduction to Psychoneuroimmunology*, Elsevier, Burlington, MA.

DSM IV, 1994, *Diagnostic and Statistical Manual of Mental Disorders*, Fourth Edition, American Psychiatric Association, Washington, D.C.

Donne, J., 1624, *Devotions Upon Emergent Occasions, Meditation 17*, in Complete Poetry and Selected Prose of John Donne, John Hayward (ed), 1929.

Erikson, E. 1963, *Childhood and Society*, Norton, New York.

_____, 1968, *Identity Youth and Crisis*, Norton, New York.

_____ , 1993, *Ghandi's Truth*,Norton, New York.

_____, 1993, *Young Man Luther, Norton, New York*

Fairbairn, W.R.D. 1952, *Psychoanalytic Studies of the Personality*, London, Routledge.

Feldenkrais, M. and Ginsburg, C., 2005, *Body and Mature Behavior*, Frog Books.

Freud, S., 1914, *Remembering, Repeating and Working Through*, Standard Edition, Vol. 12.

_____., 1915, *Mourning and Melancholia*, Standard Edition, Vol. 14.

Guntrip, H. 1969, *Schizoid Phenomena, Object Relations, and the Self*, IUP, New York.

Hazell, C.G., 1984a, "Experienced levels of Emptiness and Existential

Concern with different levels of Emotional Development and Profile of Values," *Psychological Reports,* 1984, 55, 967-976.

_____, 1984b, "Scale for Measuring Experienced Levels of Emptiness and Existential Concern," *Journal of Psychology,* 1984, 117, 177-182.

_____, 1989, "Levels of Emotional Development with Experienced Levels of Emptiness and Existential Concern," *Psychological Reports,* 1989, 64, 835-838.

_____ , *Alterity and the theory of Positive Disintegration: an organizing template.* Proceedings of Dabrowski Conference, University of Calgary, Alberta, August 2006.

_____, 2003, *The Experience of Emptiness,* Authorhouse, Bloomington, Indiana.

_____, 2005, *Imaginary Groups,* Authorhouse, Bloomington, Indiana.

_____, 2006, *Family Systems Activity Book, ,* Authorhouse, Bloomington Indiana.

_____, *2009, Alterity, The Experience of the Other,* Authorhouse, Bloomington, Indiana.

Herman, J., 1992, *Trauma and Recovery,* Basic Books, New York.

Hirsch, I, 2008, *Coasting in the Countertransference,* Analytic Press, New York.

Janet, P., *L'automatisme psycholgique: essai de psychologie experimentale sur les formes inferieures de l'activite humaine. (Paris, FelixAlcan, 1889; Paris, Societe Pierre Janet/Payot, 1973)*

Juhan, D., 2003, *Job's Body, A Handbook for Bodywork,* Station Hill Press.

Jung, C.G. 1971, *Psychological Types,*Princeton University Press.

Kast, V., 1993, *A Time to Mourn,* Daimon Verlag.

Kernberg, O., 1975, *Borderline Conditions and Pathological Narcissism,* New York, Jason Aronson.

_____, 1976, *Object Relations Theory and Clinical Psychoanalysis,* New York,
Jason Aronson.

Klein, M. 1935/1964, "A Contribution to the Psychogenesis of Manic-Depressive States," *Contributions to Psychoanalysis.* McGraw Hill, New York.

_____, 1946, "Notes on Some Schizoid Mechanisms," in *Writings of Melanie Klein, Volume 3, Envy and Gratitude and Other Works,* Hogarth Press, London.

_____, (2002) *Envy and Gratitude.* New York, Free Press.

Koch, L., (1997), *The Psoas Book,* Guinea Pig Publications.

Kubler-Ross, E., 1993, *On Death and Dying,* Scribner Classics.

Kohlberg, L., 1981, *The Philosophy of Moral Development,* Harper and Row.

Kohut, H. 1971, *The Analysis of the Self,* I.U.P., New York.

_____, 1977, *The Restoration of the Self,* I.U.P., New York.

Laing, R. 1969, *The Divided Self,* Pantheon, New York.

Lawrence, W. Gordon, *2005, Introduction to Social Dreaming,* Karnac, London.

Lopez-Corvo, R., 1995, *Self Envy,* Aronson, New York

Lowen, A., 1972, *Depression and the Body,* Penguin, New York.

_____, 2003a, *Fear of Life,* Bioenergetics Press.

_____, 2003b, *The Way to Vibrant Health, Bioenergetics Press.*

_____, 2005, *The Betrayal of the Body,* Bioenergetics Press.

Mahler, M. 1975, *The Psychological Birth of the Human Infant,* Basic Books, New York.

McWilliams, N., 1994, *Psychoanalytic Diagnosis, Guilford Press.*

Menzies-Lyth, I., 1960, *A Case Study in the Functioning of Social Systems as a Defense Against Anxiety,* Human Relations, 13: 95-121.

Maslow, A., 1968, *Toward a Psychology of Being,* Van Nostrand, Princeton.

Masterson, J., 1972, *The Treatment of the Borderline Adolescent,* Wiley, New York.

Minuchin, S., 1978, *Psychosomatic Families,* Harvard.

Montagu, A., 1986, *Touching, The Human Significance of the Skin,* Harper Paperbacks.

Myers, I., 1995, *Gifts Differing, Understanding Personality Type,* Davies-Black.

Myers, T. , 2001/2009, *Anatomy Trains,* Elsevier, London.

Ogburn, M. K., 1976, *Differentiating Guilt According to Theory of Positive Disintegration,* Unpublished doctoral Dissertation, University of Wisconsin-Madison, Counseling and Guidance.

Ouspensky, P. D., 1973, *The Psychology of Man's Possible Evolution,* Vintage.

Pelletier, K., 2003, *Mind as Healer, Mind as Slayer,* Delta.

Pert, C., 1999, *Molecules of Emotion, The Science Behind Mind-Body Medicine,* Simon and Schuster, New York.

Piaget, J., *Piaget Sampler,* ed. Sarah Campbell, Wiley, New York.

Racker, H., 1968/1982, *Transference and Countertransference,* Karnac, London.

Rank, O., 2010, *The Trauma of Birth,*Martino Fine Books.

Reich, W. 1933, *Character Analysis,* Orgone Institute Press, New York.

Rice, A.K., 1965, *Learning for Leadership,* Tavistock, London

Rogers, C. 1961, *On Becoming a Person,* Houghton Mifflin, Boston, MA.

Searles, H., 1979, *Countertransference,* IUP, New York.

Selye, H., 1978, *The Stress of Life,* McGraw-Hill.

Shapiro, F and Forest, M., 1998, *EMDR: The Breakthrough "Eye Movement" Therapy for Overcoming Anxiety, Stress AND Trauma,* Basic Books, New York.

Spitz, R., 1965, *The First Year of Life,* IUP, New York

Stern, D., 2000, *The Interpersonal World of the Infant,* Basic Books.

Sutherlin, S. and Schierl, D., 1970, "Patterns of Response among victims of Rape." *American Journal of Orthopsychiatry,* 40. p. 503-11.

Tobin, S., 1988, *The Unique Psychology of the Very Old,* Center for Gerontology.

Tustin, F., 1972, *Autism and Childhood Psychoses,* Hogarth, London

Van der Kolk, 1995, *Childhood Trauma, The Long Term Effects, (video)*, Cavalcade Productions, Nevada City, CA.

_____, (ed.), 2006, *Traumatic Stress, the Effect of Overwhelming Experience on Mind, Body and Society*, Guilford Press.

Wells, L., 1985, *The Group-as-a-Whole perspective and its Theoretical Roots.* In A. Colman and M. Geller (eds) *Group Relations Reader 2*, (pp. 109-126) , A.K. Rice, Washington, DC.

Winnicott, D. W., 1960, "Ego Distortion in Terms of True and False Self," in *The Maturational Processes and the Facilitating Environment*, pp 140-152, Hogarth, London.

_____, 1964, *The Child, The Family, and the Outside World*, Pelican, New York.

_____, 1965a, *The Maturational Processes and the Facilitating Environment*, IUP, New York.

_____, 1965b, *The Family and Individual Development*, Tavistock Publications, London.

_____, 1971a, *Therapeutic Consultations in Child Psychiatry*, Hogarth, London

_____, 1971b, *Playing and Reality*, Basic Books, New York.

Yeats, W. B., 1989, "The Second Coming" in *Collected Poems of W. B. Yeats*, Finneran, R.J. (ed), Macmillan, New York

Zimbardo, P. 2004, *Quiet Rage, The Stanford Prison Experiment*, DVD, Stanford.

INDEX

2437069R00112

Printed in Great Britain
by Amazon.co.uk, Ltd.,
Marston Gate.